Become One

Become the best version of yourself through fitness

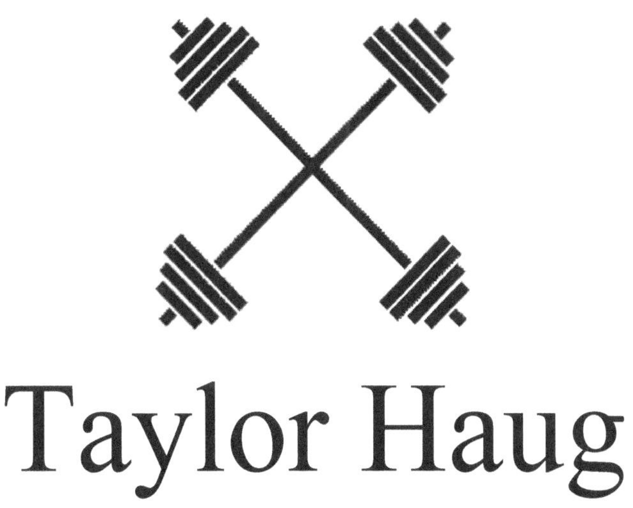

Taylor Haug

Check out the author's website at becomeonefitness.com

Be sure to follow Become One on Twitter, Instagram, and Facebook: @_become_one_

Become one, change your life

I would like to dedicate this book to my brother: the person who has had the biggest impact on my life.

Thank you Scott, you have truly changed who I have become as a person.

See you at the top.

Contents

Hear from the Become One Athletes!

Scott H: 4th Degree Isshian Ryu Black Belt, Bodybuilding Enthusiast

"I can't say enough about how Taylor and the Become One program has changed my life. I was at a point where it seemed I hit a 'plateau' in everything I was doing. From my business to body building in general, I just couldn't seem to progress in the way I wanted to and I was frustrated about it. But when I started applying the principles in The Become One program, everything changed. I smashed through the fitness plateau and added a half inch of muscle to all the major muscle groups within a short 8 weeks. My 6-pack is now showing through in great detail, which of course I'm very happy about. With the shift in my mindset, my coaching business started to bring in a record amount of income and clients. If you want to grow as a person and achieve all of your fitness goals in record time, I highly recommend The Become One program and Taylor's guidance!"

Dalton R: College Athlete, Aspiring Bodybuilder

"Before I was introduced to the Become One method of training, I figured the more weight I pushed / pulled the bigger and better results I would get. Taylor's workout philosophy transformed my entire workout routine and forced me to focus on the quality of rep versus the quantity of weight. As a college athlete, I am always looking for physical workouts to improve my physique as well as my muscle strength and conditioning. I have followed the Become One method for 6 months now, and I can honestly say that I have taken huge strides since beginning this process. I recommend Become One to every individual because you will learn to develop a mental approach to working out to receive the best outcome."

Shannon A: Former College Athlete, Accounting grad student

"Before Become One, I was very frustrated with myself because I fell out or my workout routine. School became stressful and I couldn't keep up. So I skipped a day at the gym...one day turned into two days, two days turned into a week, and before I knew it I had taken about two months off! I felt like I lost my "glow" which caused me to be down on

myself and dread going to the gym. I finally said enough is enough and contacted Taylor. Taylor and the Become One program helped me to get back into a routine that worked for me. As a student who's graduating early, working part-time, and working an internship, I wanted a routine that would fit into my busy schedule without any issues. Taylor did just that for me, and continued to work with my routine making it flexible for my schedule. Become One has done tremendous things for me to get to the fitness level I use to be at and, most importantly, allowed me to get my positive mentality back. Taylor is a coach that truly cares about each and every one of his clients. I 110% recommend his program to anyone who's looking to improve their physical self, as well as their mental mindset!"

Anthony G: High school Athlete

"Taylor and the Become One program helped not just in weight lifting, but with all aspects of my life. He was able to change my mental mindset so that I could translate that to other areas of my life, both on and off the field. He personalized a routine specifically for me that made me faster and stronger in every way. Taylor committed his full attention to my success as an athlete and made sure I was 100% satisfied with me results. I would recommend him to not just athletes,

but everyone!"

Ja'quan M: College athlete, aspiring professional basketball player

"I've know Taylor for most of my life as we grew up playing football and basketball together. These past 3 summers he has been training me and I've seen nothing but improvement in not only my basketball abilities, but my life. He's taught me to have the great mindset in anything I do in life. He has had a huge influence on the man I am today. I am 110% satisfied with my results and we ain't even done yet!" #goat

Tyler S: Successful weight loss athlete

"Before I started Taylor Haug's "Become One" training program, my body, spirit and mind were far from where I knew they could be. I tried numerous different programs, but in the end the same result; the lack of needed motivation and results. Taylor Haug has been a lifelong friend and teammate of mine, and when he reached out to me I knew this program was different. His motivation and dedication to my one on one training is something I needed to become what I knew I could be. In 6 weeks time, I smashed all goals and saw results that made me feel confident to be in my own skin once

again. Life changing is something that comes to mind every time I get home from training, and I know there are others out there who can truly succeed with this program. I'm not the best athlete. I've never been the best I could be, but now I realize this is all within my grasp. Taylor Haug's "Become One" training program is something I recommend to anyone who is trying not to just perfect their body, but perfect a new lifestyle. A lifestyle that changed me. A lifestyle of dedication, hard work and in the end results. Not just as a friend, but as a student I can't thank him enough for helping me find this lifestyle. Become One, is something I will always keep in mind and use in my everyday life not just in the weight room."

Katie L: Martal artist, tough mudder competitor

"I am a fifty-one year old woman facing her first Tough Mudder. I lacked the upper body strength needed to complete the ten to twelve mile long obstacle course. I couldn't do pull-ups or dips. I could not achieve my goals on my own. The Become One journey is challenging, but extremely rewarding. Not only did I meet my goals, I crushed them! I now believe I will be an asset to my Mudder team, not a liability. Thank you, Taylor!"

Taylor Haug: Become One Author

Think about times in your fitness life where you've wanted to reach a particular goal. Did you reach that goal? Did it come slowly over time? Did you achieve it very fast? Let's think about this for a moment. My goal, for as long as I can remember, has always been to gain weight. I've always been a skinny, thin kid. So my goal was to always put on more weight so I could gain more muscle! But for years I allowed my thoughts to dominate my results. My results were a direct reflection of my thinking. My thoughts were "This is so hard! I can't do this. Who has time to eat 6 meals a day? It's impossible for me to gain weight. I eat everything I can and still don't gain weight!" And on top of all these thoughts, I go into the gym and see myself in the mirror. I see my present self, who still hasn't gained any weight, still hasn't put on the muscle I've been looking for, and still continue to think the same thing every time I walked in the gym. Needless to say, I didn't go anywhere and I didn't achieve my goal. And because of this, I continued to make up excuses; "Maybe it's because I'm not old enough. It's all genetics, so it's not my fault. I'm in college so eating six times a day isn't possible."

Now let's diagnose the problem:

- *My thoughts were focused on what I wanted*
- *My thoughts brought me down rather thus giving me a*

negative attitude

- *My thoughts were on the present rather than on the results I wanted to achieve*

- *I would see myself as small and skinny rather than big and strong*

- *I would make excuses for myself which continued to give me negative thoughts*

- *Myself image was not where it should have been; my thoughts constantly told me I "wasn't big enough"*

Our results are a direct reflection of our thoughts. Over time I began to realize that my thoughts also have a impact on my fitness and health. So I made a connection one day: "If I'm to look the best I possibly can, then I must change my thoughts and mindset connected with working out". And from that day on, my fitness results have never been the same. I have begun to implement various techniques and strategies that allow me to keep my thoughts in check with my goals and my future self. I began adopting techniques such as affirmations, meditation, among others. Because of these techniques not only did my physique begin to change, but my mental mindset did a complete 180. These techniques have changed the way I have approached working out tremendously. And I would like to share them with you!

I promise you, if you stay true and consistent with this program, you will receive the results you want and more!

Introduction

"Are you committed to becoming something great? Or are you just interested?"

-Taylor Haug

Is this book for you?

First off I would like to commend you on picking up this book. It takes a humble person to pick up a book to improve themselves because no one wants to admit that they need help; or that they aren't where they want to be yet. But there is no shame in this, because no one has ever been able to do it alone. It doesn't matter where you are on your journey in life. An individual can always improve and be better. Even the best in history had help to become who they are. So congratulations on taking the first step towards your greatness. Let's take this journey together and create something the world has never seen.

Is this book for you? Of course! I'm happy to say that this book is for everyone. And I say that because this book isn't just about improving your body, it's much more than that. This book is going to allow you to reach out to potential that you didn't know you had, not just in fitness, but in all areas of your life. There is much more out there than what the everyday person realizes. I want you to reach out and become something you've only dreamed of, because it's possible.

Whatever goals you may have for yourself, this book is going to help you to get there. We're going to explore how to use your mind in order to achieve the best results possible. Everyone has the potential to use their mind in such a way that will allow them to reach higher potential. If the mind is in the right place, anything is possible.

So let's get started. Remember, you've already taken the hardest step, that's seeking help and knowledge to bring you to the next level. Now it's time to become something extraordinary.

What is Become One?

When I go to the gym, my mind is the muscle that's working. My physical body is the result of my mind working: I'm a sculptor shaping my masterpiece through constant thoughts of improvement.

Become One

What do you think about when you hear the words "working out"? When most people hear those words they think physical - they think changing or improving the physical body. Whether it's losing weight, gaining muscle, toning, or whatever else, it's always been physical movements that control our results. However, what if I told you that your weight loss or weight gain starts and finishes in the mind? Does this make you question your workouts? You may be thinking, *"Taylor how in the world does it start in the mind?"* Well it's simple; our results are a direct reflection of our thoughts. When one thinks weight loss, one receives weight loss. When one thinks muscle gain, one gets muscle gain. It's that simple. Your dream body will be achieved by changing your thoughts, mental mind, and your plan. It's a simple change to your workouts that will allow you to achieve more results than ever before.

What is Become One? Become One is a training program that allows you to improve everything about yourself. With this program, you will not just improve your body, but your mind and spirit as well. When most people workout, they look to improve their physical self. However, through the use of different routines and techniques, one will be able to improve more than what they think is possible. Would you like an increase in energy? How about a boost in self confidence? Or increased awareness about your body and its capabilities?

And of course, would you like to have a body that turns heads everywhere you go? Then this is the training program for you.

You will work out smart, safe, and in the most productive way possible. Results are achieved with a vision, goals, a plan to get there, and absolute consistency and persistence. The Become One program is laid out perfectly for your gain. No matter what your desired end result, I will help you get there.

Become One is going to show you how to become that person you've only dreamed of becoming. Let's go on this journey together and Become One with who we were meant to be.

Message from the author

What does it mean to be passionate about something? I believe being passionate about something means you're willing to sacrifice anything to that cause your truly passionate about. And it's only when you live that passion that you can truly say you're carrying out your life's purpose.

What do I mean exactly? People ask me all the time why I take working out so seriously. For a long time I didn't quite know what to tell them. But I believe it's because it's my number one passion in life, it's my true calling and what brings me the most happiness and fulfillment. There is no other substitute, working out is it for me. I am willing to give up and sacrifice anything to get my workouts in, day in and day out.

Why? Because, for me, working out isn't just a physical battle, it is mental and spiritual as well. It is my mental retreat, spiritual gateway, and physical battlefield all at the same time. There is no place like the gym…the smell of hard work and dedication, the sound of two 45's smashing together, the site of all people rallied together for the same purpose, to create the best version of themselves that they possibly can. The gym has done wonders for my life - wonders that I cannot describe in only a few words. Thus this book and manual has been created for your benefit. I believe everyone in the world should be able to look at themselves in the mirror and be able to smile and say "I did this, and I'm damn proud of myself for this creation". You are a creator; your mind is the sculptor, and your body is the masterpiece. Each and every day, you will use your mind to chisel the masterpiece you have been envisioning.

In order to do that, you can't do it all by yourself. Every successful person that has ever lived has had help at one point or another. Success doesn't happen for most people, not because it's not their destiny but because they don't know what to do, how to do it, and who to turn to. So I would like to commend you on taking the first step towards your greatness and success. It takes guts to ask for help and seek the guidance needed to become great. Just know that whatever you want in life is possible. Visualize what you want and then make it come to life. Let's go on this journey together and create something the world has never seen before.

Who is Taylor Haug?

Who am I? A college athlete? A black belt in martial arts? A personal trainer? An author? All of these things have helped shaped who I have become as a person, but they do not truly define who I am. I am someone who has the relentless drive to become the best at whatever I do in life. I know in my heart that no one will outwork me. Period. Am I cocky? Very far from it. It's my inner confidence that knows I will get the job done. If you give me the task of making you lose weight, we will get it done. If you want to become the best looking person on the planet, I will do whatever it takes to get you there. You can count on me to do the job, and then some. It is my job to make sure you leave the gym looking like you crawled out of hell...but at the same time having inner happiness knowing we just killed your workout and got you one step closer to your success. Your success is my success, your happiness is my happiness, and your fulfillment is my fulfillment.

For as long as I can remember, I have always been

known as the small kid. Throughout school in my early years, I was always the smallest kid in the class and on the field/court. When the name Taylor Haug was brought up in conversation, the short, skinny, small boy came to mind. And even to this day, people still remember me for who I was. But I knew this would not dictate who I was to become. To this day, I still work to prove to everyone that it doesn't matter who you are, you can look however you want. Needless to say I did not let others affect who I was destined to become.

Despite being short and small, I have always been the hardest worker. This isn't me being cocky, but after years of blood, sweat, and tears, I can truly say I have done everything in my power to be the best. Am I the best? Not yet. But at least I have been able to say that I did whatever it took to perform and look the best I possibly could. After years of slow maturation, I can say with confidence that my body is truly coming around. I know what it takes to take the step to the next level, and it is my job to help you take that leap.

I didn't always know what my life's purpose was. For a long time I questioned what my true calling in life was supposed to be. Am I supposed to become an engineer? How about an athletic trainer? But what about my passion for sports and coaching? Only the lord knows the struggle I went through over the years trying to figure out my life's calling. But somehow I think I had it deep down in my heart; my true passion that I knew would bring me fulfillment. That fulfillment for me is to lift weights and look the best I possibly can. And as a result, help others do the same for themselves. My passion consists of helping others realize their true potential in fitness. There is no greater feeling than helping someone reach their dreams and goals. I believe everyone should be able to look at themselves in the mirror and smile.

Why fail when success is an option? If everyone had the simple choice of either being in shape or being obese and overweight what would you choose? Obviously you would choose to be healthy! But for some reason a large majority of people decide to take the easy route and be unhealthy in their daily lives. I encourage you to decide to be part of the select few individuals who will do whatever it takes to become the best. Most people say they want to look better, but not everyone is willing to do whatever it takes to achieve that. Take the journey of a lifetime and become who you've always wanted to be.

Let's take this journey together because no one can do it on their own! I surely didn't do it alone. Stay with me and we will do wonders together. Stay with me and let's create a masterpiece.

"As a young man I remember being told that the guy that goes to the gym is the guy that is concerned with the physical, and the man that goes to college is a man that is concerned with the development of his mind. I struggled with that as a young man. Because they're not separate. To identify myself as a bodybuilder is to identify myself as a thinking being. My body becomes a physical manifestation of my thoughts. My power is not my body. My power is my mind. My mind is at work. To gain command of this is to gain command of your thinking, to gain control of your thinking. Is to gain control of the picture of your life."

Kai Greene
IFBB Professional Bodybuilder, 3X Arnold Classic Winner

Part I: The Core Areas of Your Life

"For me, life is continuously being hungry. The meaning is not simply to exist, to survive, but to move ahead, to go up, to achieve, to conquer."

-Arnold Schwarzenegger

Why choose Become One?

We've all heard it before: the newest machine that "guarantees" the six pack, the personal trainer who will make you the next Mr. Olympia, or the newest pill that make you shredded in 30 days. So what's different about Become One? Become One is designed to first improve your mind. If the mind is in the correct state, anything can be achieved. But if it's not, then failure is almost certainly inevitable. That's why Become One is so different compared to other workout programs. My goal is to give you the mental mindset and tools you need to be successful so that in the future you don't need my help anymore.

Let's look at the three pillars of your life: physical, mental, and spiritual.

PHYSICAL: This Become One program is not like any other personal training / personal development program. Not only will you improve your physical self, but you will improve other areas of your life as well. But let's take a look at what the Become One program will give you physically:

- Become One will help you reach your physical goals and beyond.
- This program will help you accomplish any physical fitness goal you may have; weight loss, muscle gain, toning, strength, etc.
- Increased gains in other areas such as flexibility and speed, because of what the program requires you to do on a consistent daily basis.
- Become One will give you an increase in everyday energy. Your body will feel healthy and energetic day in and day out.
- This program will put you on track to accomplish many more fitness goals in your future because of the knowledge you will receive upon completion.

- Workout injury free and stay injury free.
- Most importantly, this program will improve the way you look and feel!

<u>MENTAL</u>: Unlike most personal training programs, Become One will aim to improve your mindset and mental approach towards your fitness. Yes that's right, I said mental approach. Everything we do starts in the mind, so why should working out be any different? Let's see what mental improvements Become One can give you:

- Learn to set your own personal fitness goals and stay consistent in pursuing them.
- Become One will help you change your outlook on fitness. No more dragging workouts, it's time to get better.
- Through different exercises, your mind will consistently want to get better and achieve more with your fitness level.
- Thoughts become things: Become One will make sure that throughout your workout you think thoughts that will positively affect your workout. This means your mind-muscle connection. You will be able to connect with muscles you've never been able to see or feel before.

- Become One is going to make you feel good about yourself. Let's look in the mirror and see the person we're happy to be. Improved Self Image!
- Stress, frustration, anger? We will slowly release this energy through means of fitness. Let's live a healthy life we can feel good about.

SPIRITUAL: How can working out be spiritual? Well through this journey we will try and find who you really are! Who are you? What do you really want for yourself? Through this program, we will aim to answer these questions through fitness. Spiritual gains include:

- Finding yourself through means of fitness
- Through working out, we will clear the mind of all things; we'll focus on the task at hand: going to work.
- Creating emotional balance; controlling those highs and lows
- After the completion of the program, you will feel like you can conquer anything!
- Spiritual is also about giving; therefore as you feel better about yourself you will be able to give more to people closest to you in your life. (Spouse, kids, friends, your cause, etc.)

You have to understand that working out is much more than just lifting things up and putting them down. Working out is much more than just moving weight around while talking to other lifters. The gym is the place where success or defeat happens. Too many people walk out of the gym without feeling fulfilled or feeling like they did what they came there to do. Don't just go to the gym to go through the motions, Become One with who you're meant to be. Do you want to feel good about yourself? Do you want to be able to use what you learn in the gym in other areas of your life? Do you want to improve the life of not only yourself, but the people around you? If so, keep reading and press on. This is a lifetime journey that will make you connect with that inner being that you haven't been trained to believe in. Find out who you really are and take the challenge like so many others have.

The "Become One" way of life

All three pillars contribute to your overall success of who you become. If you'd like to become the best you can be, all three pillars must be improved

In this Become One program, you are going to follow a very strict routine. It's simple, but it doesn't mean it will be easy. One of the biggest common failures when trying to be successful in fitness is the lack of consistency (we will address how to overcome this later). You must follow the program to get the results that you want. Persistence! The key word for consistency. Every day you must work toward your goals and dreams. If you're not working at it every day, they will never be realized.

"A quitter never wins. A winner never quits."
-Napoleon Hill

In this program you will follow five simple steps to reach success:

- Vision
- Goals
- The Anatomy
- The Game Plan
- The "Education"

These five simple steps are the building blocks of your success. Each step has specific purpose. It is vital that you don't skip any steps if you want to be successful. I see many athletes jump the gun and go right to training without understanding what they would like to accomplish. You can't be the best you can be without knowing exactly where you want to go. Nothing prolongs your results more than wandering aimlessly around the gym without a purpose. The mind and body must consciously know exactly where they must head if they want the best results possible. So you must give them a direct plan of action in order to achieve the results you want.

Every step is critical to developing each pillar of your life: physical, mental, spiritual. In each step you will be improving those areas to help you reach your goals faster. Remember in order to get the best and fastest results, you must not think of this journey as just physical. You will be taking strides to your mental and spiritual self in order to make this journey a successful one.

The Become One lifestyle is a lifestyle that not everyone will live. Everyone can live the lifestyle if they choose to, but not everyone will. It's not just about going to the gym every day and training. It's about living every day with fulfillment, knowing that what you did today is going to get you to where you want to be; everyday taking another step forward towards that end goal and vision. It's not easy trying to reach the top - but if it was, then the whole world would be on top of the mountain enjoying the view.

Every great athlete completes these steps in order to see their dreams realized. Now it's your turn.

Vision

"If you can see it in your mind, you can hold it your hand."

-Bob Proctor

Before moving forward, let it be clear that in order for this program to be successful you cannot skip any step in this program. Each step is vital to becoming the best you can be. Every journey starts at chapter one…

What's your vision? I've heard "vision" as defined as "seeing your desired future as though it was already here." To some, this step may be irrelevant. However this is critical to your success. Not just in fitness, but in anything. Many people in life have sight but no vision. You must understand this true fact in order to truly know what it is you're looking for. It's not enough to just see in the now; you must visualize the results you want to achieve. You must believe and know without question that whatever your end desired result is will become realized no matter the circumstances.

It is important to not only have a vision of what your desired future is, but to also see it as if it is already here. You have to believe that what you want is already here in your possession. Believing is feeling the achievement before it has physically happened. You must feel joyful, eager, and grateful about the certain outcome you'd like to see. Why? If you are happy now you will get what you want much faster because you will put yourself in a better state of mind. If you know deep within yourself that you will get where you want to be, then there is no need to be sad and frustrated now. Be happy now and use what you have at your disposal now. This may seem absurd to some athletes, but this is crucial to your success. The athlete, who can see their desired future and believe they already have possession of it, is one step closer to success.

Let's take a look at some examples:

In today's fitness world, it can be very difficult to keep your vision in check. It's hard enough being judged from the people around you about your physical appearance, especially if you are starting far from where you would like to end up. Along with this many people are self conscious about their bodies when starting out or if they aren't seeing the results they would like to have. And here's why: when most people walk into the gym and start to workout, all they see is their current self. They take one look in the mirror, maybe in the locker room or out on the floor, and see what they look like right now. Yes it's obvious right? Obviously they see their current selves' in the mirror right? So what do I mean?

An athlete must be so consumed with their vision that it almost becomes an obsession. Consumed means to fill one's mind with, or give full attention to, one goal. If they are not consumed, they will never get to their end result. And if they do, they will get there very slowly and in a time frame that was not desired. When one looks in the mirror, they must see their vision. They must see their end result rather than who they currently are. This is why so many people get discouraged and quit. If someone is 300 lbs with a goal of reaching 200 lbs, they must consume themselves with the number 200. It must become an obsession where they only see 200 lbs rather than 300 lbs. If every time they step foot in the gym they get discouraged because they see "themselves", they will never reach 200 lbs. You must visualize and see your vision no matter the circumstances. You have to believe no matter what: "I will reach my goals".

The same goes for gaining weight and muscle. If one has the goal of reaching 185 lbs when they are currently at 160 lbs, they must consume their mind with the number 185. They must believe that they will reach that number regardless of the circumstances. They must constantly batter the mind with muscle building and weight gaining thoughts in order for them to reach their goal.

Keeping your vision in check

In order to keep your vision in check, there are many techniques you can do. I have implemented all of these and when successfully completed, the results are tremendous.

Let's take a look:

<u>Meditation:</u> Meditation is huge because it has various benefits. In this case, it affects your mental and spiritual self by allowing you to connect with you vision.. Set aside just 10 minutes a day to just close your eyes and relax; think about your vision and where you want to go. Just 5 minutes in the morning and 5 minutes at night can do wonders for your vision. Don't think about how you're going to get there, that will come. Just think about where you'd like to go and most importantly, how you would feel if you had your vision realized. This is huge! You must feel an emotional connection to your vision. Without an emotional connection, it will be hard to visualize yourself already having possession of your vision. As stated, set aside at least 15 minutes a day to meditate on what it is you want. Meditating can be done in various ways and everyone is different; I prefer to lie down and listen to instrumental music as I meditate. But again, everyone is different.

Pictures: Using pictures is a great way to keep your mind focused on where you want to go. Let me give you an example. If one's goal is to be a bodybuilder, then posting pictures of the best bodybuilders of all time around their house is a great way to keep their vision of becoming a bodybuilder. I have done this myself with great success. I would post pictures of the greats every where I could see - my bathroom, bedroom, car, etc. These "greats" would consist of Arnold Schwarzenegger (Professional bodybuilder, 7X Mr. Olympia and actor), Ronnie Coleman (IFBB professional bodybuilder, 8X Mr. Olympia) and Kai Greene (IFBB Professional bodybuilder, 3X Arnold Classic Winner). This allows you to only see people who had similar goals as you and have already achieved elite status. Another great place to put these pictures is in your gym bag or gym journal. Every time before, during, and after your workout you will be forced to see them! If your mind can visualize the end result over and over, it will know the direction to go. You must train your subconscious mind to know what it is you truly want.

Motivational Videos: Videos are a great way to keep

your vision in check. It's easy to go a week focusing on your vision. But it's hard to keep it going for 12 weeks, especially if it's your first time trying to accomplish a big goal or vision. So why not use the help of others who have been down the path you want to go? We live in a world where we can get the help of anyone using a simple source, YouTube! YouTube is a great way to get tips, advice, and motivation, all in one place. Watching videos of where you want to go is absolutely huge because you can learn from the best. Not only learn, but also get motivated when things get tough. Zig Ziglar, a motivational speaker and author, said one time "Some people say motivation doesn't last, neither does bathing. That's why it's recommended daily!" Daily motivation is sometimes crucial to keeping your vision in check. It allows you to continue moving forward just when it seems like things are too tough to move on! Some example of great motivators are: Eric Thomas, Les Brown, Tony Robbins, and Bob Proctor.

Affirmations: Affirmations may be some of the most important things you can do to keep your vision where you want it. An affirmation is the action or process of affirming something or being affirmed. In simpler terms, affirmations are really saying what you want audibly to yourself. I say affirmations daily in order to help create the image I want in my subconscious mind. Your subconscious mind cannot distinguish between what is false and true. Therefore by bombarding it with words on where you want to go, it has no choice but to think they are true. Saying affirmations before your workout (while stretching or on the treadmill for example) is a great time to do this. It will allow you to focus your entire lift on your vision.

Affirmations such as:

- "I am 165 lbs and have reached my goal weight"

- "I am strong and powerful. Every time I set foot in the gym I accomplish my goals."

- "I am a weight loss machine. Losing weight is easy for me and I can lose weight with ease."

- "I can lift any weight I choose. I am extraordinarily powerful and gain muscle every day I am in the gym."

Saying these affirmations will make your lift that much better on those days where it just seems hard to get started. Remember, in order to accomplish your dreams, you must see it as if it is already here.

We put our affirmations in the present tense because it allows us to act as if what we want is already in our possession. An affirmation in the present tense is much more powerful than one that says "I want" something. The power of "I am" is extraordinary. When you tell the mind exactly what you want in the present tense, it has no choice but to make it happen in reality.

Another point that affirmations will help with is ridding yourself of negative thoughts. People say all the time "I can't get the negative thoughts out of my head!" This is because they have not replaced the negativity with anything. If you replace the negative thoughts with positivity, the negative thoughts will diminish and go away. Fill yourself with positive thoughts and good things will come.

***An alternative to this is listening to your affirmations. For easy access, take 5 minutes and write out the results you want. Then, use a voice recorder (on your phone, app, etc.) in combination with inspiring music on in the background. While the music is playing and the recorder is on, say your new results out loud, capturing your vision in words. Listen to them while you warm up, while you're at work, driving in your car, etc. This is a sure way to make thoughts of your vision continue to bombard you subconscious mind. ***

Don't get discouraged!

I see a lot of people get discouraged because they compare themselves to the top of the mountain. We want to train ourselves to think vision, not sight. Many people have sight, but neglect to have vision! What I mean by this is too many people only see in the present and in the now. It is definitely important to see in the now, however you will never go anywhere without knowing what you want your end result to be! We want to work toward the point where you are relentless in your fight to achieve your end desired result, no matter whom or what decides to step in your way. Work on your vision continuously and it will come with ease.

Don't compare your chapter #1 in life to someone else's #20. The reason why people are at their chapter #20 in their life is because they put in the work and effort to be there. They went through each chapter to get where they are. Stop comparing yourself and saying it's impossible. It's going to take time, constant time and effort. Don't expect the overnight success. The success will come with patience, hard work, and dedication. You will get to that chapter #20 in your life by setting goals and getting there one chapter at a time. So don't get discouraged because there are people ahead of you. Stop comparing yourself and fight your own battles. "Climb your own mountain…one that is higher than anyone could ever imagine!"

How can your vision help you elsewhere in your life?

Working at a vision can help you in other areas of your life because it will teach you many different traits that are necessary to becoming successful. These traits/tools can be commitment, hard work, consistency, discipline, and focus. Each of these traits are needed in order to become the best you can be at whatever you would like to do in life. If you are successful at one vision - take fitness for example - then it will be easy to apply the same techniques implemented into other areas you would like to be better in.

If one successfully completes their fitness vision, that success can very easily be transferred to another area such as relationships, or even in your profession. It simply requires you to start the process over and focus your thoughts on a different area.

This Become One program will help you in all areas of life. Teaching an individual how to become successful in one area of their life can help them drastically in other areas. Take this program with hard work and commitment in mind and see your life begin to change.

Your vision worksheet:

What is your vision?

Write exactly what you would like to achieve and have into your possession. What do you look like? How do you feel? What have you accomplished? Start with an "I am...." statement.

____

____

____

____

____

____

____

____

What visionary steps will you take to get there? Will you use pictures, videos, or affirmations? Will you try all three?

I want you to be very specific here. State in exact words the very steps you will take to achieve your vision. For example if you'd like to use affirmations, what will you say?

____

____

How will your vision help you outside of the gym:

Will it help you at your job? Will you share your vision with others such as your family? Will it help you accomplish other goals you may have?

What are the consequences of not doing the worksheet? It's easy to read books and listen to audio books. But to actually apply the knowledge gained and learned is a whole different story. Stop what you're doing and complete the worksheet. Its three basic questions that will help you go to the next level. Completing this will put into perspective where you are right now. Completing this will allow you to see where you would like to go. We don't want to roam around, we want a clear sense of direction and to know exactly where we want to go.

Remember you cannot skip any step; every step is a brick being laid down to complete the house. If you cut corners then the house will eventually fall down. Complete each step and then move on.

"Self development is everything. At the root of my own experience (bodybuilding) comes down to self mastery. A lot of times people get caught up in how small their waist is or how big their arms are or how much they can bench. What it's really all about is controlling your thinking and focusing your concentration towards the pursuit of the end result, All anybody can do is bring their max effort to the forefront and put their best foot forward each day. Don't worry about a particular person or setback, that's not your job. Your job is to manage yourself to the best of your abilities. Focus on that and you will find that it's more impactful. Keep training, keep learning, you will evolve"

Kai Greene

IFBB Professional Bodybuilder, 3X Arnold Classic Winner

Example vision worksheet

What is your vision? Write in words exactly what you would like to achieve and have into your possession. What do you look like? How do you feel? What have you accomplished? Start with an "I am…." statement.

"I am 180 lbs of pure muscle and perfection! I have a perfect healthy body with perfect symmetry and proportion. I can push and pull any amount of weight I want which allows me to look perfect! All of my muscles, bones, tendons, and ligaments are 100% healthy which allows me to workout every day and accomplish my goals."

Or…

"I am so happy and grateful now that I have reached my goal my goal weight of 160 lbs! I feel fantastic! I am happy and healthy, this is the best I have ever felt! I continue to lose weight at a rapid rate and look absolutely perfect!"

What visionary steps will you take to get there? Will you use pictures, videos, or affirmations? Will you try all three?

I want you to be very specific here. State in exact words the very steps you will take to achieve your vision. For example if you'd like to use affirmations, what will you say?

"In order to reach my vision, I will start to say affirmations

every day. I will do this first thing in the morning before I start my day so that I am in a positive mindset and ready to tackle anything that happens throughout the day. I will say five simple affirmations:

- I am content and happy!

- I am my goal weight of 160 lbs!

- I am healthier than ever; all of my muscles, bones, tendons, and ligaments are 100% healthy!

- I have the best body in the world and it gets better every single day!

- I am perfect and will reach my goals in record time!

I will say these affirmations every single day for 30 days!"

How will your vision help you outside of the gym: Will it help you at your job? Will you share your vision with others such as your family? Will it help you accomplish other goals you may have?

"My vision will help me outside the gym because I am much happier about where I am! I'm making strides in the right direction and because of that, my attitude and mindset has changed completely. My personal life at home is much better and continues to improve every single day! My family notices much more energy in me and I am a positive influence for everyone at the house."

Or…

"My vision will help me outside of the gym because it will help me accomplish other goals I want to set for myself. I can go through the same process I did for my body vision for things like finances and my relationships. It's the same exact process! I just have to switch around the wording and the other areas of my life will improve right along with everything else!"

These are just examples of what an individual may write. Everyone has a different vision so take some time to think about it and put it in your own words. Don't be afraid to write whatever comes to heart, there is no right and wrong! When I write out my vision I write a good amount, almost a full page to cover all three questions. But do what is needed for you.

Goals

"Set your goals high and don't let anyone hold you back. If you truly believe you can achieve something, you can do it. Don't let anyone turn your sky into a ceiling."

-Taylor Haug

This next segment is absolutely crucial to this program. It's about setting up your goals. What are goals? Goals are the end desired result or stepping stones one looks for when focusing their energy and power on that result. Goals are so important and are often overlooked. But when goal setting is properly done, it can change the way you workout and propel you further than you ever thought possible.

Goals are going to be your stepping stones in order to reach your dream and vision. Setting up proper goals is what will propel you to your end desired result, if done properly. If goals are not set up properly, one will become discouraged and fail to make continuous progress. Visions can be very big, especially if they have been one's dreams for so long. This is why it is necessary to set goals. Without goals, one will not have any way of reaching that vision. If a person has a vision of making 1 million dollars but has no plan of action and is without "stepping stones", they will never get there! You must understand that visions do not get accomplished overnight. One may get "lucky" every now and again, but in order to achieve long lasting results and see them constantly, one must set up goals. You must set up stepping stones in order to be successful.

Why do people fail to accomplish goals they have set for themselves?

A huge problem with fitness today is that too many athletes don't create goals for themselves. When a person wants to improve and get better, but doesn't have a clear vision of exactly what they want, their progress will be slowed or even stagnated. The mind must have a clear path of where to go if it's to get better. Without goals, the mind is essentially lost! In this program, you will be making goals for yourself so that you can envision exactly where you want to go with your health and fitness.

Some athletes make goals, but never achieve them.

Why does this happen to so many athletes? Well there are many reasons for this failure. But one of the biggest is the failure to remind themselves of their goals. The mind needs to continually be reminded of where you want to go. How many people do you know have made goals but have quit after the first two weeks? Or better yet, they don't even remember the goal they set for themselves. This is because they are so used to what they have been doing; they revert to "their old thought process". If the mind does not get taken over by the vision, it will revert to old habits and soon the goal will be lost. I know from personal experience that if I don't constantly see my goals throughout the day, they will be forgotten in a week. In order to avoid failing to see my goals, I have implemented various techniques that allow me to stay on track and keep my mind focused on my vision. I have used these techniques personally. They will make an impact, but you must stay consistent with them or else you will fail.

All of the techniques used are simple and easy. It takes no grueling work to do this. They are simple and easy but extremely effective. The more you see your goals, the faster and easier you will achieve them. But remember, a goal without a plan is just a dream…

Goal techniques

<u>**Goal Card:**</u> A goal card is a small card, such as an index card, that has your goals listed on it. On one side of the card, your goals will be listed, along with the time frame you'd like to accomplish them in (date which you'd like them to be completed, example "March 1st 2017"). The goal will be written in the present tense just like your affirmations. On the opposite side, something personal such as a meaningful quote will be written. This card will be brought with you everywhere! I have seen people put this card in there wallet, that way, every time they open it up they see it. Some people just put the card in their pocket and take it out every so often to look at it. What I do personally is I tape the index card to the back of my phone. I have found that this is the most effective way to remind myself of your goals and dreams. It's very simple, but the results from this can be tremendous. The thing we touch most throughout the day is our cell phone. Therefore this forces me to see my goals numerous times every day whether I want to see it or not! Below is an example of a goal card that can be used:

<u>Setting Up Reminders:</u> As stated earlier, many athletes neglect to look at their goals. Not because they don't want to, but because they just simply forget. They haven't developed the habit of looking at their goals yet. Setting up reminders is a great way to eliminate this problem. I set up reminders on my phone to go off every day, three or more times. I set alarms at different times throughout the day (morning, afternoon, night) so it will force me to turn them off after I see the message.

<u>Print-outs:</u> Another useful technique is printing out your goals on paper. Once multiple copies have been printed, they will be posted up everywhere; your bedroom, bathroom mirror, in your car, office, refrigerator, etc. Doing this technique will help you see your goals wherever you are. However, this only works for some people. I have found for me this only works for so long. After a period of time, my eyes and body become accustomed to the print-out and I begin to overlook it. But it is all about personal preference and what works best for you.

<u>Writing out your goals:</u> This may be the most effective way to reach your goals as quickly as possible. It's simple, but I have found it to be the most effective. I take an empty journal (I label this my goals journal) and use it specifically for my goals only. Every day I write one page, then continue on every single day. I write out my goals as though I have already accomplished them. For example, if my goal is to reach a goal weight of 185 lbs, then I write out the goal as if I have already reached it. I may write something such as: "I am so happy and grateful now that I have reached 185 lbs because I look and feel great. I can press and pull incredible amounts of weight which allows me to look perfect. I am strong, vascular, and perfectly proportional!" I will do this with each one of my goals. I do this extensively so that I fill up one page per day. Now you don't have to writ as much as I do, but that's what works for me.

Time Frame

Another reason why people fail to reach their goals is the time frame they set for themselves. Many people make goals but never achieve them because the time frame of their goals is too long. For example, when January comes around, people all across the nation will make New Year's resolutions and goals. But what happens by the time May comes around? They have forgotten about their goals and they go down the drain! To eliminate this, it's crucial that you keep your goal time frame small. Weekly goals, monthly goals and 12 week goals, are all good examples of how to eliminate "forgetting" your goals. Yearly goals are very good if you have been goal setting for years and years. But even the best sometimes have trouble being successful at them. You must find what works best for you because everyone is different.

As a personal example, I would make a habit of making yearly goals for myself. Not just in fitness, but in all areas of my life. But when the end of the year came around only a few of my goals have been completed. What I did not understand was the time frame of my goals was hindering my results. There was no focus of power and no urgency to get them done because I had a full year to accomplish them. In order to get better results I switched up the time frame and focused my power on only a couple of goals at a time. Once the switch was made, the results were almost instantaneous. I was urgent about completing them and was able to focus my energy and power on what I needed to do. This problem can be known as hyperbolic discounting. Hyperbolic discounting refers to the tendency for people to increasingly choose a smaller-sooner reward over a larger-later reward as the delay occurs sooner rather than later in time. The farther away a reward is in the future, the smaller the immediate motivation to achieve it.

Find what works best for you and stick with it. This is crucial if your vision is to be reached. Don't wait around for years, waiting for the results to come to you. Make those goals and attack whatever it is that you want. With this approach, you will be there in no time.

Lack of desire

Lack of desire may be the most common among the people who fail to accomplish their goals. Why? Because it is easy to be average and mediocre. It sounds harsh but it's the sad reality in today's world. Most people are comfortable with average, or comfortable with being "comfortable" so they stop striving for greatness. One must be comfortable with being uncomfortable; this is the only way to get results. Why? Because you start to experience the growth you need to attain your goal. The change in vibration of your body is what makes you feel uncomfortable. Reaching beyond what you think is possible will propel you past your goals and allow you to achieve your vision and dream.

As the great motivational speaker Eric Thomas once said "you must be allergic to average". There is no better way to put it! In order to be the best you must push past the average and mediocrity in today's society. Look past all fear and all doubt, and accomplish what you were born to accomplish.

You have what it takes inside of you; find the desire within yourself because no one is going to find it for you. No one is going to do the work for you and no one is going to tell you what you must do. Don't become another statistic, become something great. Become One with yourself and push beyond what everyone thought was possible.

Applying goals to the rest of your life!

Goals are good for all areas of your life. You can apply what you do in the gym at work, at home, in your finances, and in your personal life. People make goals because they are unsatisfied with their current circumstances and they want to get better. Therefore you can do this with anything you want to get better at. Once you understand how the whole goal process works, you will be addicted to it. Why? Because goal setting works! Once you set a goal and accomplish it for the first time, there is no better feeling.

So why not apply this to other things as well? Improve your relationships at home. Improve your financial situation. Improve your whole life by creating what you have envisioned in your head, because it's all possible with proper planning, goal setting, and action.

Your goals worksheet

Write out two fitness goals you'd like to achieve. We're going to start with 2 goals because it will not be overwhelming. If we start with too many, it will be hard to accomplish if you're just getting started. Let's focus on two things you truly desire and get there first!

These can be anything you'd like to achieve in your health! Ex.) I will achieve 160 lbs, I will lose 10 lbs, I will cut out pop from my diet, or I will go to the gym 4 times a week.

Notice I start the goal with "I will" not "I want". "I will" is much more powerful than "I want". "I will" says that I WILL ACHIEVE IT when "I want" is just a mere wish saying I might get there.

1.) ____

____

2.) ____

____

Now let's take a look at the time frame that you'd like to accomplish these goals in. You must be careful about what you choose because often it's the time frame that dictates whether you are successful or not.

If the time frame is too short, you cut yourself short on time. If you stretch out the time frame too far, it's easy to become lazy and get off task.

Your time frame can be anything from a week (if your goal is to "lose 3 pounds this week" for example) to 8 weeks (if your goal is to "gain 2 inches on my quads" for example) to 12 weeks (if your goal is to finish a certain workout routine for example).

Review your goals and make the best choice you can. I recommend using the same time frame for both goals as it will make it easier to track.

Time frame for my goals is:

I will have achieved_____________________________(i.e losing 10 pounds) by _______________(the date you want to achieve your goals) which is ______________________________________ .
(i.e 8 weeks from now, one week from now, 30 days from now)

Next let's take a look on how you will accomplish these goals! There are several ways that were listed to help you stay on track to accomplishing your goals.

Write out the techniques you will use to stay focused on what's important to you. State exactly what you will do in order to stay on track, be specific. Will you use the goal card? Will you use printouts? Where will these be placed? BE AS SPECIFIC AS YOU CAN!

I WILL…

____

____

____

____

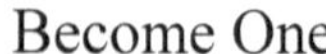

____

____

____

____

After these goals have been successfully accomplished, just repeat the process! Keep doing the process until your vision has been realized. Now this make take months and years to finish, but in the end your vision will be realized and if you truly want it bad enough it will all be worth it.

I can tell you from experience that there is no greater feeling than accomplishing a series of goals. If the dream you set out to accomplish means something to you any, small amount of labor or work to get there will be worth it. Keep working and don't settle. What you truly want won't be easy to accomplish. But think about it, if what you truly want was easy to achieve everyone would already have it…and if that was the case the process wouldn't be as fun!

Example goals worksheet

Write out two fitness goals you'd like to achieve. We're going to start with 2 goals because it will not be overwhelming. If we start with too many, it will be hard to accomplish if you're just getting started. Let's focus on two things you truly desire and get there first!

These can be anything you'd like to achieve in your health! Ex.) I will achieve 160 lbs, I will lose 10 lbs, I will cut out pop from my diet, or I will go to the gym 4 times a week.

Notice I start the goal with "I will" not "I want". "I will" is much more powerful than "I want". "I will" says that I WILL ACHIEVE IT when "I want" is just a mere wish saying I might get there.

1.) I will be 160 lbs OR I will lose 10 lbs

2.) I will lose 4 inches on my waist OR I will have a size 28 waist

Now let's take a look at the time frame that you'd like to accomplish these goals in. You must be careful about what you choose because often it's the time frame that dictates whether you are successful or not.

If the time frame is too short, you cut yourself short on time. If you stretch out the time frame too far, it's easy to become lazy and get off task.

Your time frame can be anything from a week (if your goal is to "lose 3 pounds this week" for example) to 8 weeks (if your goal is to "gain 2 inches on my quads" for example) to 12 weeks (if your goal is to finish a certain workout routine for example).

Review your goals and make the best choice you can. I

recommend using the same time frame for both goals as it will make it easier to track.

Time frame for my goals is:

I will have achieved *my goal weight of 160 lbs* by *September 1st, 2017* which is *8 weeks from now.*

Or..

By *September 1st, 2017* I will have achieved *my goal weight of 160 lbs* which is *8 weeks from now.*

Next let's take a look on how you will accomplish these goals! There are several ways that were listed to help you stay on track to accomplishing your goals.

Write out the techniques you will use to stay focused on what's important to you. State exactly what you will do in order to stay on track, be specific. Will you use the goal card? Will you use printouts? Where will these be placed? BE AS SPECIFIC AS YOU CAN!

I WILL…

"To stay on track with my goals, I will use a goal card and printouts. I will print out my goals on 8 sheets of paper and place them up around my house. I will place these in my bedroom, my bathroom, my car, and my kitchen so that I see them every single day. I will also use the goal card and place it on the back of my phone so that I see it when I use my cell phone."

Part II: The anatomy

"I am a believer that we shape and create the life we choose and I believe that the tool we have to do that is our mind."

-Kai Greene

Your body

In order to have the best body you possibly can, you must know your body inside and out. What are the best exercises for each body part? Which exercises do what? How do I know which order to my exercises in? This is what this section is for. I will be going over each body part and talking about each different exercise so that you can accomplish that end goal you want to achieve.

Chest

The muscles of the chest are:

- pectoralis major

- pectoralis minor

- clavicular pectoralis (upper chest)

The chest is one of the biggest muscles in the body. Therefore the chest must be hit from all angles in order for it to fully develop. Many people say they want a "big chest". But what is really needed is a chest that is symmetrical and proportional throughout. For example, the upper chest is lacking on most novice lifters because they spend too much time on flat bench and don't vary the angles. Vary the angles as much as you can and it will help you develop that chest you have envisioned.

There are six basic exercises that are generally done to work the chest. They are:

- **Flat barbell bench**

- **Incline barbell bench**

- **Flat dumbbell bench**

- **Incline Dumbbell bench**

- **Flyes (multiple variations)**

- **Dips**

These exercises listed here are the major exercises to increase your chest development and strength. Of course there are others not mentioned, but these are the best core exercises for your chest.

Flat bench presses: Often this is done at the beginning of the chest workout or upper body workout because it is a compound movement. Also, it is the exercise generally that we like our chest to be fresh for. On flat bench, we would like all muscle fibers on deck so we can push as much weight as we can (correctly that is). Barbell and dumbbell are both great to do. I encourage you to do both as switching it up will allow you to recruit different muscle fibers in the chest. For example, dumbbell is much harder as you go heavier because of the supporting muscles needed to press up two separate weights. Both are crucial to perform if you want great chest development.

Incline bench presses: As I stated earlier, this may be a great place to start your workout if your upper chest is lacking. Most lifters jump right on the flat bench because they want to lift the whole gym right from the get go. However, if you assess your weaknesses and realize you need more development in your upper chest, I encourage you to start your chest workout here at the incline. Remember it's not always about the weight; it's about creating the best balanced body you can. A balanced and proportional body is the best looking body and what we want to shoot for.

Flyes: Flyes are one of the best exercises for overall

chest development. Flyes allow you to get a great stretch and contraction that you may not get while doing regular pressing movements. Flyes can be done with lots of variations. However, chest flyes are one of the most wrong performed exercises. If done incorrectly, you risk serious injury or just recruiting the wrong muscles to move the weight. Hence why many novice lifters front delts overpower their upper body. However, if done correctly, chest flyes will serve you well in your chest development. There are several variations you can perform, they are: flat dumbbell flyes, incline dumbbell flyes, cable flyes (upper lower, and middle), the pec deck machine, and pectoral fly / rear deltoid machine. If you're a novice lifter, I suggest using machines to start in order to get the proper mechanics. Remember it's not always about the weight, especially with flyes. Get a full stretch and a full contraction.

Dips: Dips can be done for either chest or triceps. They can be great for chest development because you can be sure to get a full stretch and contraction which we sometimes miss with our other pressing movements. These dips can be done with added weight, or just bodyweight. I personally like doing strictly bodyweight when it comes to dips for chest because I can focus hard on contracting my chest, rather than other muscle groups such as my triceps. If you add too much weight, it becomes an "up and down" movement rather than a slow stretch and squeeze. If you're a novice lifter, I recommend holding off on these for some time, until you gather some chest development, as it's a tough exercise to master. A novice lifter may not be able to contract the targeted muscle group; in this case it's the chest.

Each exercise listed is great for chest development. Experiment with new exercises and see what your body responds to the best. Everybody's body is different and will react differently. Therefore, what works well for me might now work well with the next person, and so on. Along with this, everyone's weaknesses are different. Assess your body and decide what is needed to make yourself the best you can possibly be.

Back

The back is composed of:

- the traps

- the rhomboids

- the lats

- the spinal erectors (lower back)

- the teres

The back is composed of lots of different muscles. Lots of different exercises must be performed in order to hit every muscle group throughout the back. From the traps and rear delts, all the way to the "Christmas tree" composed in the lower back: every muscle must be accounted for.

To have a fully developed back, there are seven core exercises that you should perform. They are:

- **Pull ups**

  Lat pull down (with variations)

- **Dead lift**

- **T bar row**

- **Seated row**

- **Barbell row**

- **Pull over's**

Of course there are tons more back exercises one can perform to gain back development. But these are the best movements to gain a nice thick back.

Pull ups: Pull ups may be the best bodyweight exercise one can perform. Although fairly tough if you are a novice lifter, the pull up will give you huge strength gains especially if you use a strong mind-muscle connection. The pull up can take large amounts of time to master. It's easy to just go up and put your chin on the bar and go back down 10-12 times. But what's tough is having a good mind muscle connection which allows you to focus on the lats, traps, and rhomboids while performing the exercise. A good way to make huge strength gains is adding weight while performing this exercise. Once the exercise becomes easier, adding weight can keep the challenge for the advanced lifter. However don't add weight too soon or else it will be inevitable for you to recruit other muscles more such as your biceps and forearms for example. (Just like the dips that we talked about earlier)

Lat pull downs: The lat pull down is a fantastic exercise because it can be done in many different ways. With the use of different grips and attachments, different muscles in the back can be targeted. The lat pull down is also a great way to work on the mind muscle connection with your back because it can be tough to do so with pull ups. Some variations you can perform are wide pronated grip, regular supinated grip (chin ups), close grip with neutral grip, and behind the neck pull downs. Behind the neck pull downs are sometimes frowned upon because it puts stress on the rotator cuff. However, they can be hugely beneficial if they are done with a hard contraction and squeeze, rather than lots of weight. Keep the weight light and contract hard through your traps and rear delts for example. Of course when going heavy the lat pull down can be great because you can lock yourself in and focus just on pulling. Whichever workout routine you may be doing, the lat pull down can be used for huge strength gains.

Dead lift: My outlook on dead lifts is much different

than most people. I stay away from heavy barbell dead lifts because they can be strenuous on the lower back joints, and here's why: a lifter may put 405 on the bar, and slam the weight back and forth thinking that he's stimulating lots of muscle fibers. He/she may be stimulating lower back fibers, but what they don't realize is the stress they are causing. Jolting heavy weight on and off the floor can be hugely strenuous, especially when you're not controlling the weight but rather having it bounce on and off the floor. I'm not saying it's bad to do heavy weight with dead lifts because of course it can be beneficial. But I do a slightly different variation to help stimulate more fibers in my back. It's the dumbbell dead lift variation. The dumbbell dead lift takes out the jolt of hitting the weight on the ground at the bottom, forcing you to control the weight through the whole movement. Controlling the weight throughout the whole movement stimulates more muscle fibers because there is no point of rest, you must work at every point during the rep. You can still go very heavy with this variation, strap in with some heavy dumbbells and build that "Christmas tree".

T bar row and barbell row: I put these two together because they are similar movements. Both are great for development of a thick back. Both can help with the v-taper we are trying to develop. I recommend wearing a weight belt when going heavy with these exercises as they will put large amounts of stress on the lower back. But if done correctly, they will do wonders for your development. The T bar is one of my personal favorites. I personally like to load the T bar with 25 lb plates rather than 45 lb plates because with the smaller weights I can get more ROM (range of motion). This especially helps with the development in the lower back. More ROM means more stretching and contracting of the muscles in my back, which means more development.

Pull over's: I personally like the pull over machine rather than dumbbell pull over's, especially if you're a novice lifter. It can be tough to contract the targeted muscle with dumbbell pull over's, therefore the machine can be a great place to start. But make no mistake about it, whether you're an experienced bodybuilder or just getting started, machine pull over's can be an absolute killer exercise for your lats. Mind-muscle connection is key to keeping the stress on the back and not the arms or chest. This exercise is great for bodybuilders because it's a great way to work on your lat spread pose. At the bottom of the movement, making your lats as wide as possible and flexing hard just like you're doing a lat spread pose can really serve you well.

It is very important to have a strong back as it is labeled as one of the biggest stabilizers in your body, especially your lower back. Along with this, back injuries are among the most common injuries in today's world. Training properly and safe is key when training the back. Train hard, but be sure to train the right way.

Legs

The muscles of the quad are:

- vastus medialis

- vastus lateralis

-vastus intermedius

The muscles of the hamstring are:

- biceps femoris

- semitendinosus

- semimembanosus

Yup, it's that time...legs! Not everyone has love for legs, but it is absolutely crucial to train legs just as much as your upper body. Why? Well of course it makes your body look proportional by giving you the classic physique look (the x shape). But training legs, believe it or not, will also help you with other areas of your training. If you're an athlete, then legs might be the muscle group you need to train the most out of any other muscle group. It's hard to train legs, trust me I know it's not easy. But training legs will make you a better lifter in the end, and make you look 100x better by giving you proportion and symmetry.

Let's look at the core leg exercises first, then go into calves later. The main leg exercises are:

- Squat (back and front squat)

- Leg press (leg sled)

- Walking lunges

- Hack squat

- Leg extensions

- Leg curl (lying or seated)

- Stiff legged dead lift or Romanian dead lift

These are the core exercises to build strong, thick legs. As I said, they are not easy, make no mistake about it. But get in the gym and get it done.

Squat: Squatting is the number one leg exercise. Why? If done correctly, it's the best compound movement to perform because your able to hit every muscle group in the leg: quads, hamstrings, and glutes. There is much discussion, and always will be as far as I'm concerned, with the form and depth of the squat. Everyone has a different opinion when it comes to squatting. Do you go past 90 degrees? Do I have to squat heavy to build big muscles? Do I lock out my knees at the top of the movement? These are just some common questions that one may ask when squatting. I'm sorry to say there is no "real" answer to any of these questions. Everyone's body is different and responds to different stimulants. Personally, I do what works best for my body, which means going past 90 degrees isn't necessary. This also means I don't lift huge amounts of weight when I squat. But again, this is my personal preference. When you look at a guy like Ronnie Coleman (8x Mr. Olympia), lifting heavy weight was his way of life and what worked best for his body. On the other side of the spectrum, you have a guy like Kai Greene (4x Arnold Classic winner) who believes a strong contraction paired with good mind muscle connection is the basis for muscle building which means you don't have to lift the whole gym. Find what gives your leg muscles the most stimulant and stick with it.

Leg press: Every lifter has his/her own preference for different exercises. For me, leg press is my personal favorite because I can load the sled up with weight without having to worry about straining my back in the process (unlike squatting if your form isn't the greatest). I don't have much flexibility through my hips (I'm working on it!), which means it's tough for me to take my lower back out of the equation when I squat. Of course I still squat, but I just keep the weight lighter than what I do on the leg press. The leg press is also good because, with different foot positions, you are able to hit different muscle groups. With a close stance, you can crush the quadriceps. With a slightly wider stance, the inner thigh and hamstrings are able to get the work.

Walking Lunges: I like walking lunges over stationary lunges because walking adds extra tension which makes you work much harder. Walking also works balance and the support muscles surrounding your leg. This is a great movement to work inner thigh development as well. Keep the weight light and squeeze through your glutes and hamstrings. As the rep range gets higher and you get tired, your quads have no choice but to work. Great all around exercise.

Hack squat: Hack squats are another great compound movement. Regular hack squats are great, but if you want to take it up a notch then take a look at a video of Tom Platz doing hack squats as he gives hack squats a slightly different variation. Enough said on this subject.

Leg extensions: Great exercise for the quads. Doing extensions will allow you to have great development throughout your whole quad, especially when done till failure. Lots of sets, lots of reps, lots of volume. No secret with extensions, pump up the volume and get to work.

Hamstring curls (seated and lying): Hamstring curls can be done either seated or lying. I personally like lying better because you can get a better stretch through the hamstrings. And with lying you are able to activate your glutes. Both are great for hamstring development and should be done every leg day. A superset I often like performing is starting on seated curl for 20 reps to pre-fatigue the muscle, then immediately jumping onto the lying leg curl for another 20 reps, but this time focusing on the slow stretch and contraction of the muscle. Give it a try!

Stiff legged dead lift or Romanian dead lift: This a good exercise for hamstring and glute development. However if done wrong, the tension can be put on the lower back instead of the leg muscles. If this is the case for you, drop the weight until the form is mastered. Don't worry, if it is done correctly, light weight will still give you great development through your hamstrings. Remember, a good stretch and strong contraction is the basis for good muscle building.

Included in legs training is calves. Calves cannot be overlooked; they are the foundation for your legs and, if not trained,, then your lower half will not be in proportion. Arnold Schwarzenegger used to have small calves in comparison to his legs, here's how he got rid of the small calves.

"When I first came to America (in 1968), I didn't have big calves. In 1969, I visited Reg Park at his home in South Africa and stayed with him for a while. He would get up at 5 a.m. to

train. So Reg, being my early idol, I got up at 5 a.m. to train with him. The first thing he did every session was 10 sets of calf raises. His calves were a huge 20 inches. I looked at them and said, "I want calves like that." So he put 500 pounds on the machine and started his first set. I screamed, "Five hundred pounds! I'll rip my Achilles!" He told me, "When you walk, with one foot in mid stride, the other foot is supporting 250 pounds, so both feet can support a 500-pound workload. To really make the calves grow, you have to go up to 1,000 pound calf raises." I said, "No way!" In one year my calves grew two inches. They grew so quickly that some people began to say I had gotten calf implants. They would check them out, looking for any scars when I flexed them. I took it as a great compliment that my calves had improved so much—they eventually got to be 21 inches— that some people thought I had implants."

The muscles of the calf are:
- the gastrocnemius
- the soleus

There are two muscles that make up the calf. They are the soleus and the gastrocnemius. In order to hit both muscles, two different calf exercises must be done. They are:

- Standing calf raise

- Seated calf raise

You must do both exercises if you want to hit both muscles. Why? The soleus is a deep muscle that lies underneath the gastrocnemius and it's much harder to hit. Therefore when we perform seated calf raises, the gastrocnemius is relaxed because the knee is bent and allows us to hit the soleus head on. The gastorcnemius is what is mostly seen in aesthetic terms. But a strong soleus will make the calf look larger by propping up the gastrocnemius.

A great way to perform calf raises is the 10/10/10 method. This consists of doing 10 raises with the toes in and heels out (which allows you to hit the outside of the calf), 10 raises with the feet parallel (which allows you to hit the middle of the calf), and 10 raises with the toes out and heels in (which allows you to hit the inside of the calf). Most lifters calves are not proportional throughout; personally mine are still on there way to full development. Years of walking and running a certain way will develop the calves you have today. This rep scheme will allow you to hit all areas of your calf and bring out the proportion that is desired.

Shoulders

The 3 parts of the shoulder are:

- anterior deltoid (front delt)

- medial deltoid (side delt)

- posterior deltoid (rear delt)

The shoulders are a unique muscle because they work much more than any other upper body muscle. Why? Because when every upper body part is being trained, the shoulders work too! This is especially true for novice lifters whose form isn't correct. Taking a look at the bicep curl, most beginner lifters perform this wrong because they incorporate a lot of their front delt while doing the exercise. Another example is with triceps press downs on cables; novice lifters tend to push also with their shoulders instead of lightening the weight and keeping the tension on their triceps. I could go on all day but that isn't the point. The point I would like to make is to take a look at your shoulders and see where your weakness lies. For many, their medial and posterior deltoids lag behind their anterior (for many their side and rear deltoids lag behind their front). This obviously doesn't happen intentionally. But as I stated earlier, the shoulder works in more ways than we realize and therefore works certain muscles more than others over time. So evaluate your shoulders and determine where your weakness lies and start your shoulder workout there. This is a bit unorthodox, but if you want your shoulders to be equally proportional then this is what needs to be done. The weakness needs more work to be on the same level as your strength.

Let's take a look at the core shoulder exercises:

- **Standing shoulder press (barbell or dumbbell)**

- **Seated shoulder press (barbell, dumbbell, or machine)**

- **Shrug (barbell, dumbbell, machine)**

- **Side lateral raise**

- **Front raise**

- **Upright row**

- **Rear delt raise (dumbbell or machine)**

- **Behind the neck lat-pull down**

These are the best exercises to build big round shoulders. We can call them boulder shoulders! Again, hit your weak areas first. This will allow your shoulders to be equally proportional throughout and equal on all heads.

Shoulder press: The shoulders press is the best overall shoulder exercise one can do. It really helps to build mass and builds muscle in all three heads depending on the type of press you perform. The shoulder press can be done several different ways as listed: standing, seated, barbell, dumbbell, machine, smith machine, behind the neck, and in front of the neck. Each different press will put tension on a different part of the shoulder. For example, a behind the neck shoulders press will allow you to get development in the rear delts whereas a press in front of the head will put the tension more on the front delt. Personally, I make sure I mix up my pressing movements to hit my shoulders from all angles.

Shrugs: The shrug is the best exercise for your traps if you want to build mass. Shrugs can be done in various ways: barbell, dumbbell, smith machine, in front of the body, or in the rear of your body. Just like shoulder press, each different shrug will help development a different part of the trap and shoulder. Doing too much of one exercise will make a different part of your muscle more developed than another. It's crucial to do various different movements to keep the symmetry and proportion.

Side lateral raise: The side lateral raise is the primary movement for the medial head of your deltoid. However this is a common exercise that is often done wrong. In this movement, it's critical to lead with the elbows and pinky. Why? When leading with your elbow and pinky, the stress and tension will be put on the side and rear of your delt taking the front out of the movement. As I stated before, our front delts get lots of work. We want to develop round shoulders that are proportional throughout. These lateral raises can also be done several different ways: standing dumbbell, seated dumbbell, one arm cable, one arm dumbbell, or machine raises. Remember; lead with the pinkies up to help development round proportional shoulders.

Front raise: The front raise is a primary movement for the anterior part of your deltoid. I typically do these towards the end of my workout because I like to hit the other parts of my shoulder first. For me personally, my front delt has better development than the rest of my shoulder, so I can give less attention to this area. This isn't true for everyone but it happens to be so for me. Ways to perform this exercise are: standing dumbbell, standing barbell, seated dumbbell, and standing cable.

Upright row: The upright is a great compound movement for the overall development of your entire shoulder. When done correctly, this exercise will work your side and rear delts as well as your traps. The same principle applies here as with side raises; lead with your elbows and try to get your elbows above your hands. This will allow for tension to be brought into the medial head of your delt. Upright rows can be done several different ways: barbell, cable machine, dumbbell, rope cable, and also with the EZ bar. In this category I also like to throw in face pulls. The upright row and face pull are very similar and tend to work the same muscles in the shoulder. Face pulls can be done on a cable machine by using the rope attachment and pulling straight towards your face, activating your rear delts and traps. Keep the elbows in line with your forehead to help activate your rear delts even more!

Rear delt raise / rear delt machine: This is my personal favorite exercise for developing the rear delts. When done correctly, this exercise will really round out your shoulders which are strongly desired by many bodybuilders. I like to perform these on the "reverse chest fly machine" instead of dumbbells. The reason being is that the machine will keep your form perfect every rep, when with dumbbell form tends to get sloppy towards the end of the set. This exercise can be performed on the reverse chest fly machine, seated with dumbbells, or standing with dumbbells.

Behind the neck lat pull down: Yes, that's right behind the neck lat pull downs. "But Taylor I thought the lat pull down was a back exercise?" You are right. But when done slightly different, you can take the tension off of your back and place the tension on your rear delts and traps. The exercise should be done with light weight; light weight will allow you to focus on the mind muscle connection between your mind and your traps/rear delts. To some this might be a tough exercise because many are used to doing this movement for back. Drop the weight and focus on a good stretch and contraction.

A big focus should be placed on the rear delts and traps because in order to create the desired v-taper in your back, your upper back must be fully developed throughout. Many novice lifters concentrate on the big movements like pull ups and dead lifts but don't place enough emphasis on the upper back. Focusing on these areas during your shoulder workouts will allow you to be fully developed from top to bottom.

Biceps

The muscles of the biceps are:

- the biceps brachii

- the biceps brachialis

Everyone's favorite subject...BICEPS! Of course biceps are fun to train. I mean who doesn't like an insane arm pump? But with that being said, often times biceps are trained improperly. In my opinion the bicep curl is the main exercise that is done wrong. Novice lifters who grab 40 lb dumbbells and swing them up and down stimulate their ego more than their biceps. The bicep needs to stretch and contract in order to grow. When most lifters do dumbbell curls, there is no stretch. The elbow must bend to stretch the bicep muscle. If the bicep never fully stretches, that means the front delt is probably getting most of the tension during the movement, hence why I said earlier that many lifters front delts are often times over developed. As is stated, the bicep must stretch and contract with every exercise.

The main biceps exercises are:

- Barbell curl (or EZ bar)

- Dumbbell curl (standing or seated)

- Preacher curl (dumbbell or machine)

- Hammer curl (dumbbell or cable)

- Reverse curl (barbell, dumbbell, or cable)

The best way to train arms is lots of volume: lots of sets and lots of reps. You want to pump as much blood into the muscle as possible. Hit the biceps from all angles and get a great muscle pump.

Barbell curl: The barbell curl is the biggest mass builder for your biceps. As stated with any biceps exercise, the biceps must stretch and contract. Of course there is a time and place for heavy weight. If you're an advanced lifter, then to get over plateaus and humps, cheat reps and heavy weight are sometimes necessary. But be sure to have a balance of both. Because if the biceps curl is done improperly too much, other muscle groups will be working more than the targeted muscle. The barbell curl can be done with a barbell, an EZ bar, or with cables.

Dumbbell curl and hammer curl: Your bicep is composed of a short head and a long head. The dumbbell hammer curl will work the long head of the bicep while the basic bicep curl will generally hit the short head. To create well developed biceps, both heads must be hit each time you do arms training. These two exercises can be performed with dumbbells standing or seated. An alternative to dumbbell hammer curl is doing it on the cable machine with the rope attachment.

Preacher curl: The preacher curl is the best exercise to create the desired high peak on the bicep. The preacher curl works the short head of the bicep creating the "mountain" we all desire. Generally, genetics dictate what your biceps will look like. But doing preacher curls will hit the short head head on and create higher peaks. The preacher curl can be done various different ways: machine preacher, barbell preacher, and single arm preacher. Also in this category are isolation curls, such as the one arm concentration curl and two arm cable curl. The one arm concentration curl can be performed while seated with your elbow on your inner thigh. The two arm cable can be performed by using two handles on the cross over cable machine and squeezing into a "double biceps" pose.

Reverse curl: The reverse curl hits the brachialis really well in the biceps; the muscle that helps the biceps pop. The reverse curl is a good biceps exercise, but it's also good for the forearms. While doing this exercise, if you take your palms and face them down while performing the exercise the emphasis will be put on your bicep and the bottom of your forearm. But if you take your palms and point them out at the top of the movement, the bicep and top of the forearm will get the work. This exercise can be performed with: a barbell, an EZ bar, dumbbells, or a cable.

Remember training arms isn't too tricky. When training arms, concentrate on lots of volume with lots of reps and sets. Be sure to hit both heads of the bicep; the long head and short head.

Triceps

The three heads of the triceps are (triceps brachii muscle):

- the medial head

- the lateral head

- the long head

When people think of big arms, they mostly think of big biceps. However the triceps accounts for most of the arm thickness because it is a bigger muscle than the biceps. The triceps contain three muscles, while the bicep contains only two. Therefore if you want big arms you must work the triceps just as hard. Don't think of just high peak biceps, but rather a full arm that contains a defined horseshoe in the tricep and also a thick bicep. Again, arms aren't tricky to train; lots of sets and reps is what is needed to build thick full arms.

The main triceps exercises are:

- Dips (machine, bodyweight, and weighted)

- Cable press downs

- Skull crushers (dumbbell or machine)

- Overhead extensions (dumbbell or cable)

- Close grip bench press

In order to develop the best triceps possible, all three heads must be hit. So it is critical that various different exercises be performed.

Dips: dips are the best mass builder for thick full triceps. These can be done on a machine or on dip bars. If you're a novice lifter, I recommend doing machine dips because it will be easier to keep the focus on the triceps rather than the chest. If you're advanced, then doing either can be extremely beneficial. Weighted dips on the dip bars are a great exercise, but of you go too heavy then it can be tough to keep the focus on the triceps. Choose whichever works best for you to get the best triceps contraction. Remember, it's arm day, which means we want to work our arms not our chest. Don't get heavy and sloppy. Focus on good form and work the targeted muscle.

Cable press downs: Cable press downs are also another good mass builder, depending on what type of attachment is being used. A straight bar, EZ bar, or V bar will help with mass building. Load up the weight and contract the triceps hard at the bottom of the movement. However if an attachment like a rope is used, it's going to work the triceps a bit differently. The rope is going to help develop the desired "saber tooth" that is present on a lot of developed lifters. Therefore using the rope is going to help with definition rather than mass building. With the rope, lighten the weight and focus on a hard contraction.

Skull crushers: Skull crushers can be done is various ways: dumbbells, straight bar, EZ bar, or on a machine. For mass, I like to use an EZ bar or straight bar. But using dumbbells will allow you to get a longer stretch of the muscle. Both will with the triceps a bit differently; doing various different types will allow for the best triceps development. A quick note for skull crushers: keep your elbows in while doing the movement. If the elbows begin to flail, then your shoulders will begin to do the work. If your elbows begin to flail, that typically means you're doing too much weight and should lighten.

Overhead extensions: Overhead extensions are critical to do every arm workout because they hit the long head of your tricep otherwise known as the "under-hang" of the arm. These can be done in various ways: two arm dumbbell, one arm dumbbell, EZ bar, straight bar, and on cables. Be sure to stretch behind your head as much as possible to get a full triceps contraction. Short, choppy movements won't get the job done. Stretch all the way down to the bottom of the movement to develop the best arms you possibly can.

Close grip bench press: Close grip bench press is also a great mass builder. This exercise will also help your regular benching as well. Your chest and triceps are both pushing muscles; therefore they are a catalyst for each other. Strong triceps will help your chest movements and visa-versa. This movement is tough for some people because of the angle your wrists are forced to be at. Put your hands as close together as you can comfortably, and keep your elbows in tight to your body to focus on the triceps development. This movement can be done with: a barbell, on the smith machine, or even with dumbbells. I like to do this movement superset with skull crushers. I do my skull crushers, then immediately after use that same weight and do close grip. It's a great superset and really blasts the triceps with lots of volume.

Be sure to hit all three heads of the triceps to get full development. Lots of reps and lots of volume.

Abs and core

The abs are composed of 4 main muscles:
- the serratus
- the obliques

- the rectus abdominis (upper abs)

- Lower abdominals

Abs can be trained every day. I personally train abs every time I go to the gym to train, which is typically five to six days a week. I give my abs work every single day but it's not grueling ab work daily. Usually what I tend to do is stick with a simple ab circuit and do a 2-3 sets. If I was only training my abs 3 days a week, then I would bump up the intensity. However, since I give them work every single day I keep the volume low. The big key with abs, or with any muscle, is be sure to get a full stretch and squeeze of the muscle. Your abs consists of lots of different muscles and they cover a large area. Therefore it is crucial to stretch and contract the whole muscle group. Many lifters stick with basic crunches and do not do them properly. It consists of short choppy movements with no purpose; neck movement, no hard contraction, etc. Basic crunches can be a great exercises, but only if they are done properly. Remember, stretch the targeted muscle, and contract the targeted muscle hard.

There are about a thousand different abs and core exercises, but these are my personal favorites that have given me the best results:

- Ab wheel

- Body twists

- Weighted rope crunch

- Leg raises (on bench, pull up bar, and on floor)

- Decline sit up (weighted or bodyweight)

- Basic crunches

- Side oblique's crunch (with dumbbells or on floor)

Weighted double crunch

I usually pick 3 or 4 of these exercises and put them in circuit ever day!

Ab wheel: I love the ab wheel because it's one of the best stretches for your abs. It allows you to get a full stretch from your upper abs all the way to your lower. It's also a great lower back exercise. Your lower back and abs work together as your main core muscles. Therefore it is crucial to develop them both the best you can. The ab wheel is also good because you can gradually work your way into it. If you cannot go all the way to the floor with your nose yet, then just go as far as you can. No matter how far you are able to go, it still makes you work. As you get stronger, you can slowly progress your way to a full stretch.

Body twists: Body twists are a simple exercise, but very effective when done correctly. Grab a weightless bar, like a broomstick, and hold it on the back of your neck in a relaxed position (like you about to press it over your head for a shoulder press). Then take your abs and suck tuck them in as much as possible like you're doing a vacuum pose. Rotate as much as you can to one side, then go to the other, back and forth in succession all the while holding your waist in. Don't go too fast, just keep a nice pace. I usually do this exercise first in my abs circuit to get my abs warmed up. Stick with high reps here, about 30-50 reps, sometimes even up to 100 reps.

Weighted rope crunch: Abs need gradual resistance just like the rest of your muscles do. If you want carved abs, then you can't just do bodyweight exercises, you must add in weight. Weighted rope crunch is one way you can do this. I like this exercise because you can do regular weighted crunches, or you can mix it up and do alternating weighted crunches where you touch your right elbow to your left knee and vice-versa. You can do this exercise standing or kneeling on your knees.

Leg raises: Leg raises are going to be your number one exercise for chiseling you your lower abs. However they can be tricky if you're not focusing on the muscle being targeted. It's easy just to move your legs up and down and use your lower back to help. But if you're truly locked in on your lower abs, this exercise is the key for that shredded look. You want to try and take all your other muscles out of it - your lower back, your legs, etc. Focus your mind on using your abs to lift up your legs, slowly and with control, with a hard contraction at the top. This exercise can be done lying down, on a pull up bar, or on a bench. You can also incorporate weight with this. But remember, if you go too heavy, other muscles will start to be recruited to get the weight up, so keep it light.

Decline sit-up: The decline sit up is a great way to get a full stretch of your abs. The angle of the decline doesn't have to be anything too steep to get a good stretch and contraction. The purpose of the decline is to make your abs work much harder, as you are going past the usual 180 degrees you are at with regular crunches. These can be done with weight, but again don't go too heavy. No need to grab 100 lb's to do a weighted sit up. Grab a medicine ball or a plate that's around 10-15 lb's and that's all the resistance you will need.

Basic crunch: Yes that's correct, basic crunches! If done correctly basic crunches can still be one of the best exercises to do. It all depends on how hard you contract you abs at the top of the movement. This is a great exercise to finish off in your circuit because your abs are already pre-fatigued making them that much harder.

Side oblique's crunch: I love this exercise because it can be tough to hit your obliques with certain exercises. This exercise can be done on the floor by lying on your side and crunching your elbow and knee together, with a hard contraction of your oblique. Or it can be done standing up with a dumbbell in one hand and crunching hard with your oblique.

Weighted double crunch: This is my personal favorite because it hits your entire abs, from your lower abs all the way to your upper abs. This can be done without weight, but it's not as effective. If you can't use weight quite yet, then start with bodyweight and work your way up. Start by lying on the floor with your feet straight out and your hands straight out. Then while keeping your arms and feet straight, crunch up and touch them together at the top of the movement, taking your shoulder blades off of the floor. Contract your upper abs and lower abs together hard at the top. Then lower them back down without setting your feet on the floor. To add weight, put a dumbbell in between your feet and hold either a medicine ball or weighted bar in your hands. Remember, don't add too much weight because your lower back will be forced to work, keep it light and contract hard.

Work on chiseling your abs every day and they will come. Be sure to hit every area of your abs when doing them. This means upper, lower, the obliques, and the serratus should be hit every time. Stay consistent and keep working even when you're sore. Doing abs while you're sore will help the soreness to go away. Remember, you are a sculptor; you can create anything you'd like to create. Chisel out that perfect body that you have envisioned in your mind.

The importance of understanding

It's important to understand that you must know your body and how it works and develops. Everyone could use a little help getting started. But there comes a certain point where you won't need help anymore because you will know your body better than anyone. That's my goal as a trainer. I don't want to train you forever! I want to give you the tools and building blocks you need to grow and understand yourself. So knowing all of this anatomy is very important because you will be able to visualize exactly what you want to look like while you are training.

Continue to study and understand yourself so that you can become exactly who you'd like to be.

Part III: The Game Plan

"A goal without a plan is just a wish."

-Antoine de Saint Exupery

Planning your success:

After you find your vision and make your goals, it's time to come up with a plan that will bring you the best results possible. Before you can take action, it's crucial to build the right plan that will move you forward, not keep you complacent. Each athlete's body will respond to different routines and it's critical to find out what works best for you.

Most routines or personal trainers want you to just lift heavy weight. However, with the Become One program, we will be building your mind-muscle connection in order to help build more muscle and burn fat faster. With any athlete, if you are able to "connect" with your muscles better, it will make you that much stronger. In some of the programs listed, they start with a "building phase". This means that for the first couple weeks of training, we will be focusing on that mind-muscle connection rather than on the weight.

We start here for multiple reasons:

1. We must learn our body before we start putting large quantities of weight on the bar. In order to get the best results possible, the body must learn how to work the proper muscle group.

2. This will help prevent injury in the future. Starting with lighter weight will help our bodies become accustomed to lifting the weight we want. This will also help work muscle groups and different parts of the muscle that we don't usually work. Because of the hard contraction, different muscle fibers will be activated thus resulting in an easier muscle contraction in the future.

3. Whether you're a beginner or expert, starting with lighter weight and a heavier contraction will still result in muscle growth. There is a common misconception with weight lifting that you have to lift heavy weight in order to build muscle. This is not true. With an intense hard contraction, the muscle will still be stimulated to activate large amounts of muscle growth, regardless of the weight being used.

4. It doesn't matter who you are, mind-muscle connection can always be improved. The better you can contract your muscles, the more muscle fibers that can be activated to stimulate muscle growth.

Once the mind-muscle connection is established, the weight and volume will be increased to build as many muscle fibers as we can. Any great weight lifter will tell you, the mind-muscle connection must be established in order to achieve the greatest results possible.

There are several plans listed as you read. If you already know your body from lifting experience, then disregard the following sentence. But I strongly suggest you start with the first plan and work your way to the next plans from there, as the plans go in order of increasing difficulty. Don't jump right to the end because it will be useless. You must get your body adjusted to such stress before moving on. Again, if you are already experienced, then assess your vision/goals and pick the right plan for you. Every athlete will be different and will respond differently to different routines. It's crucial that you find what works best for you in order to get the best results possible. I have experimented for years with different routines and exercises. Now I know what my body will respond the best with. Experiment, learn, and then execute.

The Warm-up:

Before we get into an example routine, I would like to explain a distinct difference with Become One. With the Become One Program, there is a huge emphasis on working out in a healthy way. As stated earlier, we aim to lift injury free and stay injury free. This is huge in the world of fitness. Nowadays, injuries are almost inevitable, especially when lifting as heavy as possible. However with this program, those injuries will be significantly decreased through various techniques and exercises. We will reduce the frequency of injuries without sacrificing muscle gain. With Become One, you will lift hard, but smart.

Many people associate a warm up with their physical body. But this warm up should be a warm up for your mind and spirit as well. The warm up is a time to get your mind ready for the task at hand and get rid of all other thoughts that may hinder your workout. Your workout should be completely dedicated to the bettering of yourself. You should not be worried about anything else in your life - a break up, your work problems, money, etc. Thus the warm up should allow you to clear your thoughts about everything that is irrelevant to the bettering of your body. This is crucial. If your thoughts are not completely dedicated to the improvement of your health and fitness, your workout will be brought down to a lower level.

Too many people walk into the gym and just get after it. However, I would encourage you to get yourself prepared before lifting. I cannot stress enough how much this simple warm up has helped my body. Do it with a purpose and a goal in mind, and good things will happen. I have been able to lift for the past couple years injury free. This has allowed me to get the best muscle gain I could possible get. A body cannot get better if it is sidelined. So take the warm up to heart, learn to love it, because it will make you all the better.

Regardless of the routine you perform, you will do the same warm up. I cannot stress enough the importance of the warm up. It might be tedious and long, but the benefits are tremendous. Various aspects of your fitness will increase because of the warm up. Stay consistent and the results will show.

Here is what the warm-up consists of:

- **Warm-up**

This consists of doing 10 minutes on an inclined treadmill, step mill, bike, etc. This is not a cardio session. The purpose of this is to warm up your entire body. Warming up the entire body reduces injury and allows your muscles to get ready for the task at hand. Most importantly, this is the time to get your mind ready for the lift your about to have. Time to think about the muscle group you're working that day, and to release all negative thoughts from your mind. During this time, I like to listen to specific tracks in order to help me get into a meditative state. Maybe a motivational video, or a certain genre of music. The choice is up to you, it's all personal preference.

- **Abs and core**

Abs are done every day. Abs are done before the lift to help warm up the core and back. You use your core for every exercise you do while lifting. Therefore it is crucial to get it warmed up before taking action. A couple of plans have been made up just for you, encompassing a wide variety of exercises for all goals and skill levels. This will not be grueling since it will be done daily, but we will chisel away at those abs every day. If you want the best abs in the business, you got to give them a little treatment every day. This may seem absurd to many people, but this method is often overlooked. Lots of volume to get you to where you need to be, and fast

- **Full Body Stretch**

This is absolutely crucial! Stretching every day will reduce your risk for injury, reduce soreness in your muscles, and give you increased flexibility. Increased flexibility is greatly overlooked when working out. Many people focus on the weight rather than on the contraction of the muscle. The more flexible an athlete is, the more he/she can contract the muscle or connect with the muscle group being targeted. Increased flexibility is also huge for athletes; jumping higher, running faster, better agility, are all products of stretching every day.

- **Lastly, the everyday exercises. For the ADVANCED LIFTER ONLY, you will do pull-ups/lat-pull down and dips every single day.**

A huge part in becoming stronger is being able to contract every muscle in your body. Doing dips and pull-ups everyday will allow you to work on that connection and contraction with your back as well as your chest. It is crucial to be able to contract these muscle groups because they are 2 of the biggest muscle groups in your body. With your pull-ups, you will work on the contraction with not only your lats, but your rear delts, traps, rhomboids, etc. With the dips, we will aim to push with our chest, not our triceps. This means flaring the elbows a little more and bending over to target the chest. Full stretch and full contraction with each set performed.

IMPORATANT NOTE! *Each set should not be grueling. You perform the amount you need to get warmed up and to get a good contraction. If 6 pull ups is what you need to do, then do it. Others may want to perform 10 or 12, that's okay. My personal routine consists of doing 3 sets of each, 10 reps a piece. Quick and easy.*

The Warm-up should take about 25-30 minutes, no longer. This may seem like a long time to many people. But what are the consequences of not doing it? What suffers if you don't perform this warm up? What happens if I skip one warm up one day before I lift? You have to think, if I do this warm up now then in the future I won't have to take time off for injuries and soreness. The warm up time is worth it. You will feel better, perform better, and look better. I would much rather take the time now to almost guarantee a better performance and longevity, than to skip it and rush through my workout.

It is not grueling and should not deplete you for your actual workout. Sets are minimized and limited, therefore the warm-up will warm you up, not tire you out. Stay consistent with this and the benefits will reveal themselves in time. Personally, this warm-up has allowed me to not only stay healthy for an incredible amount of time with no injury, but also to achieve huge muscle gains. As stated, every participant will do this warm-up. Regardless of your fitness goals or custom plan made for you, this is what you will do first, every time you step in the gym.

Abs Plans

I would advise to start at the top first, then work your way down after several weeks and months of training. In order of difficulty:

Core Plan #1, BEGINNER: Complete 2 sets

1.) Regular crunches: 20 reps

2.) Alternating elbows: 20 reps

3.) Lying leg raises: 20 reps

Core Plan #2, BEGINNER: Complete 2 sets

1.) Ab ball crunch: 20 reps

2.) Machine Sit-up/crunch: 20 reps

PLEASE NOTE: every gym will have some sort of crunch or sit up machine. Find which works best for your purposes. Select a light to moderate weight, and focus on the contraction.

3.) Body twists (standing with broomstick): 30 reps

Core Plan #3, INTERMEDIATE: Complete 3 sets

1.) Body twists (standing with broomstick): 50 reps

2.) Ab wheel: 10 to 15 reps

3.) Hanging leg raises: 10 reps

4.) Hanging knee raises: 10 reps

Core Plan #4, INTERMEDIATE: Complete 2 sets

1.) Decline sit-up with med ball: 25 reps

2.) Standing oblique Crunch: 15 reps each side

3.) Lying leg raise on bench: 15 reps

4.) Regular crunches: 25 reps

Core Plan #5, ADVANCED: Complete 3 sets

1.) Body twists (standing with broomstick): 50 reps

2.) Weighted rope crunch: 20 reps

3.) Weighted decline sit-up: 20 reps

4.) Weighted hanging leg raise: 20 reps

Core Plan #6, ADVANCED: Complete 3 sets

1.) Regular crunches: 100 reps

2.) Body twists: 100 reps

3.) Plank hold: 1 minute

As stated earlier, abs will be done every day. Therefore I would advise you start with the beginner plans, and work your way up. This is not going to be easy. But if you want results, you have to push your body beyond its limits. Your abs will be sore, but it's important to push past the soreness. Pushing past the soreness will push he blood and lactic acid out of the area and help it heal. Keep working every day, and the results will come.

Insight

I have personally done each of these workout plans and can tell you from experience that each plan will help you get bigger and stronger. Trust the process and be willing to try new things. Too many people don't grow, or stop growing, because they have "black and white" thinking; it's either this way or that way, and that's it. Be willing to take a leap and try something that has the potential to make you great.

Let's take a look at some example routines. Routines will vary for each person and athlete. Listed are six routines to help you build muscle. Each varies in time and difficulty. As stated these are just various examples of routines you can complete to gain as much muscle as possible:

The Beginning of Perfection

Example routine #1, after daily warm-up

This first routine is the beginning of perfection. It's a routine that has been designed for someone who is not very experienced and needs a routine to help jump start their working out career. This routine will not be as grueling and tough as the others, and will not take as much time out of your day/week. However make no mistake, it is not a cake walk.

In this Become One program example:

- 6 week program
- Weight train 3 days out of the week, with 2 days of cardio (this only requires you to go the gym 3 days a week)
- Workouts are about 60 minutes including lift, warm up,

and abs. This also depends on your focus level, so no talking or other funny business

- Workouts in italics are supersets (Do both together. For example if front and side raises are super setted, this means you do front raises first, then side raises upon finishing, without a break. Once both exercises have been completed, then rest. Then repeat for the designated number of sets.)
- AMAP means "as many as possible"

The work load in this program is toned down for the beginner lifter. If you are not experienced I would recommend starting with this program first before proceeding to the other programs. This workout should not be long, get in the gym and get it done.

Don't forget this lift still incorporates your daily warm-up. Despite which program you choose, the daily warm-up should be done before lifting. This will help you build muscle and lose fat quicker.

Training split:

Monday: pushing (Chest, Shoulders, Triceps)

Tuesday: cardio

Wednesday: lower body

Thursday: off day

Friday: pulling (Back and Biceps)

Saturday: cardio

Sunday: off day

Monday's Routine: Chest, shoulders, and triceps

1.) Chest Press Machine: 20, 15, 10

2.) Chest Fly Machine: 20, 15, 10

3.) Pushups: AMAP x3 sets

> *** If you cannot perform regular pushups, there are two alternatives. You can either put your hands on a bench to make them easier, or perform them on your knees. ***

4.) Seated Dumbbell Shoulder Press: 20, 15, 10

5.) *Front Dumbbell Raise: 10, 10, 10*

6.) *Lateral Dumbbell Raise: 10, 10, 10*

7.) Dip Machine: 20, 15, 10

8.) *Single Arm Dumbbell Kickback: 10, 10, 10*

9.) *Dumbbell Overhead: 10, 10, 10*

Tuesday's Routine: Cardio

*** Today's routine is up to you. I recommend at least 30 to 45 minutes of cardio. This can consist of using gym cardio equipment such as treadmill, bike, elliptical, stepper, etc. Or your cardio can consist of active activity such as aerobics, recreational activities like basketball or swimming, etc. Every person will have their personal preference when it comes to cardio. But the important thing is you find what brings your body the best results, as well as what you enjoy. If you don't enjoy your cardio, you will dread it every week and therefore lack the results you'd like to achieve. ***

Wednesday's Routine: Lower Body

    1.) Leg Press: 20, 15 ,10

    2.) Quad. Extension: 20, 15, 10

    3.) Lying Hamstring Curl: 20, 15, 10

    4.) Step Ups (body weight or with dumbbells): 20, 15, 10

        *** If bodyweight is easy, then add dumbbells in order to increase the difficulty. ***

    5.) Walking Lunges: 20, 15, 10

    6.) Seated Calf Raise: 10, 10, 10, 10

    7.) Standing Calf Raise: 10, 10, 10 ,10

Thursday's Routine: Off day

    *** It is very important to take off days and allowing your body to recover and heal. This is especially huge for a lifter who has just started to workout. Your body is not used to being under such stressful workouts, therefore it is vital to take rest. If you are sore, then there are many things you can do in order to reduce that. Stretching is a great way to help reduce soreness. Also, heat application, such as hot showers or soaking in a hot tub. A foam roller will also do the trick! Take today, rest up, and be ready to get back at it tomorrow. ***

Friday's Routine: Start Back, then Bicep's

1.) Pull ups: 10, 10, 10, 10

> *** Pull ups are a tough exercise. Therefore if you cannot perform pull ups, substitute one of two things, either an assisted pull up machine or lat pull down machine. Each is a great alternative. ***

2.) Seated Row: 20, 15, 10

3.) Dumbbell Dead lift: 20, 15, 10

4.) Upright Row: 20, 15, 30

5.) Straight Bar Curl: 20, 15, 10

6.) Dumbbell Hammer Curl: 20, 15, 10

Saturday's Routine: Cardio

*** Today's routine is up to you. I recommend at least 30 to 45 minutes of cardio. This can consist of using gym cardio equipment such as treadmill, bike, elliptical, stepper, etc. Or your cardio can consist of active activity such as aerobics, recreational activities like basketball or swimming, etc. Every person will have their personal preference when it comes to cardio. But the important thing is you find what brings your body the best results, as well as what you enjoy. If you don't enjoy your cardio, you will dread it every week and therefore lack the results you'd like to achieve. ***

Sunday's Routine: Off day

*** It is very important to take off days and allowing your body to recover and heal. This is especially huge for a lifter who has just started to workout. Your body is not used to being under such stressful workouts, therefore it is vital to take rest. If you are sore, then there are many things you can do in order to reduce that. Stretching is a great way to help reduce soreness. Also, heat application, such as hot showers or soaking in a hot tub. A foam roller will also do the trick! Take today, rest up, and be ready to get back at it tomorrow.

Climbing the mountain!

Example routine #2, after daily warm-up

This is the next training routine in the cycle. It consists of a little bit more volume, but were still not at the top. In this Become One program example:

- Train 5/7 days of the week, with one day off on Sunday. This requires 4 days at the gym.

- Workouts are about 1 hour 30 minutes depending on focus level, no talking or funny business. You can get this done in 90 minutes if you work and go to the gym to do what you need to do.

- 6 week program

- Workouts in italics are supersets (Do both together. For

example if front and side raises are super setted, this means you do front raises first, then side raises upon finishing, without a break. Once both exercises have been completed, then rest. Then repeat for the designated number of sets.)

- AMAP means "as many as possible"

Training split:

Monday: chest and triceps

Tuesday: off day

Wednesday: back and biceps

Thursday: cardio

Friday: upper body

Saturday: legs

Sunday: off day

Monday's routine: Chest and triceps

1.) Incline barbell bench: 20, 15, 10, 8, 6

2.) Flat barbell bench: 20, 15, 10, 8, 6

3.) *Dips for chest: 4 sets of 10*

4.) *Incline fly's: 4 sets of 10*

5.) Dumbbell overhead triceps press: 20, 15, 10, 8

6.) Close grip bench: 20, 15, 10, 8

Tuesday's routine: Off day

Wednesday's routine: Back and biceps

    1.) *Smith machine deadlift: 20, 15, 12, 10*

    2.) *Smith machine bent over row: 20, 15, 12, 10*

    3.) Pull ups: 4 sets of 10

    4.) Face pulls: 20, 15, 10

    5.) Upright row: 20, 15, 10

    6.) EZ bar curl: 20, 15, 12, 10

    7.) Preacher curl: 20, 15, 10

Thursday's routine: Cardio

You can choose your cardio. Running, doing a rec sport, swimming, biking, yoga, sprints, group classes etc. (as stated in the previous routine example).

Friday's routine: Upper body

    1.) Dumbbell incline chest press: 20, 15, 12, 10

    2.) Seated barbell shoulder press: 20, 15, 12, 10

    3.) Dumbbell side raises: 3 sets of 10

    4.) Rear delt raise/reverse fly machine: 20, 15, 10

    5.) Dips: 4 sets of AMAP

    6.) Dumbbell curl: 20, 15, 10

Saturday's routine: Legs

    1.) Leg extensions: 20, 15, 12, 10

2.) Seated leg curl: 20, 15, 12, 10

3.) Lying leg curl: 20, 15, 12, 10

4.) Leg sled: 12, 10, 8, 6, drop set

5.) Single leg squat: 20, 15, 10 (each leg)

6.) Standing calf raise: 4 sets of 20

7.) Seated calf raise: 4 sets of 20

Sunday's routine: Off day

THE MUSCLE GAINER!

Example routine #3, after daily warm-up

This example routine is for someone looking to put on muscle and get into their top physical shape. It's an 8 week program designed in a specific way to make you put on as much muscle as possible in a safe and healthy way.

Weeks 1-4 are the most important part of the routine. In these four weeks, we will be strictly focused on the contraction of the muscle. This means that the weight does not matter! I'll say it again: the weight used is completely irrelevant. We will aim to use a weight that is sufficient for us to focus on the contraction of the muscle being targeted. It doesn't mean we use 5 lb for everything, but if 5 lbs is what needs to be used to do the exercise right then so be it! We will be adding muscle because of the intense contraction with each muscle. There is no wasted movement. We will not be adding weight just make the movement sloppy, and not just be moving weight. We will be contracting the targeted muscle.

Weeks 5-8 is when we will turn up the volume. After four weeks of learning to contract the muscle at hand, we will load the bar and pump your body up with as much volume as possible. This will force your body to react in an astonishing way. Because your muscle knows the contraction, it will react 2X better because now we will be loading the bar with weight. More weight = more muscle growth. However, without the first four weeks of contractions, your muscles would not respond in the same manner.

In this Become One program example:

- Train 6/7 days of the week, with one day off on Saturday
- 8 week program
- Workouts are about 1 hour 30 minutes to 2 hours total including lift, warm up, and abs. This also depends on your focus level, so no talking or other funny business
- Workouts in italics are supersets (Do both together. For example if front and side raises are super setted, this means you do front raises first, then side raises upon finishing, without a break. Once both exercises have been completed, then rest. Then repeat for the designated number of sets.)

- AMAP means "as many as possible"

This routine does start on Sunday. If you would like to switch up the days and start on Monday instead, no problem! Switch it up to make it best for you and your schedule.

Weeks 1-4, these weeks are strictly dedicated to focusing on the contraction. WEIGHT DOES NOT MATTER.

Training split:
Sunday: chest
Monday: back
Tuesday: legs
Wednesday: chest
Thursday: shoulders
Friday: arms
Saturday: off day

Sunday: Chest
1.) Barbell Flat Bench: 20, 15, 12, 10, 10
2.) Barbell Incline Press: 15, 12, 10, 10
3.) Flat Dumbbell Flyes: 20, 15, 12, 10
4.) High Cable Flyes: 20, 15, 12, 10

5.) Machine Flyes: 15, 15, 10, 10

6.) Decline Bench: 20, 15, 12, 10

Monday: Back

1.) Lat-Pull Down: 20, 15, 12, 10

2.) Lat-Pull Down (palms toward, chin up): 20, 15, 12

3.) Neutral Grip Lat-Pull Down: 20, 15, 12

4.) Seated Row: 20, 15, 12

5.) One Arm Row on bench: 20, 15, 12

6.) T- Bar Row: 20, 15, 12, 10

7.) Dumbbell dead lift 20, 15, 12, 10

Tuesday: Legs

1.) Standing Calf (toes in, toes out, parallel): 3 sets of 10 in each foot position, **30 TOTAL REPS EACH SET**

2.) Seated Calf: 3 sets of 10 each foot position, **30 TOTAL REPS EACH SET**

3.) Calf Raise on Leg Press: 3 sets of 10 in each foot position, **30 TOTAL REPS EACH SET**

4.) Lying Hamstring Curl: 20, 15, 15, 10

5.) Straight Leg Dead lift: 20, 15, 15, 10

6.) Walking Lunge: 10, 10, 10

7.) Quad Extension 20, 15, 10, 10

8.) Squat: 20, 15, 15, 10

Wednesday: Chest

1.) Dumbbell Flat Bench: 20, 15, 12, 10, 10

2.) Dumbbell Incline Press: 15, 12, 10, 10

3.) Incline Dumbbell Flyes: 20, 15, 12, 10

4.) Low Cable Flyes: 20, 15, 12, 10

5.) Machine Flyes: 15, 15, 10, 10

6.) Pull overs: 20, 15, 12, 10

Thursday: Shoulders

1.) Smith Seated Press: 20, 15, 12, 10, 10

2.) Barbell Shrug: 15, 15, 12, 10

3.) *Dumbbell Side Raise: 15, 15, 12, 10*

4.) *Dumbbell Front Raise: 15, 15, 12, 10*

5.) Reverse Fly Machine OR Rear Dumbbell Raise: 20, 15, 15, 10

6.) Rear Press (Behind Head): 20, 15, 10

Friday: Arms

1.) Cable press down, Palms up then palms down: 20, 15, 15,10

2.) Straight Bar Curl: 20, 15, 15, 10

3.) Close Grip Bench Press: 20, 15, 15, 10

4.) Incline Dumbbell Curls: 20, 15, 10

5.) *Triceps Kick Back: 20, 15, 10*

6.) *Isolation Curl: 20, 15, 10*

7.) EZ Bar Skull Crushers: 20, 15, 15, 10

8.) Machine Preacher Curl: 20, 15, 15, 10

Saturday: Off day

Weeks 5-8, workout switches. For four weeks we focused on the contraction, contracting the muscle we're supposed to. Now it's time to load the bar. As heavy as possible, with lots of volume, while still contracting the targeted muscle.

Training split:

Sunday: chest and back

Monday: arms and shoulders

Tuesday: legs

Wednesday: chest and back

Thursday: arms and shoulders

Friday: legs

Saturday: off day

Sunday: Chest and Back

1.) Barbell Flat Bench: 20, 10, 8, 6, 4

2.) Lat-pull Down: 20, 10, 8, 6, 4

3.) Barbell Incline Press: 10, 8, 6, 4

4.) T-Bar Row: 12, 10, 8, 6

5.) *Flat Dumbbell Flys: 15, 12, 10*

6.) *One-arm Dumbbell Row on Bench: 15, 12, 10*

7.) *Machine Flyes: 15, 12, 10*

8.) *Seated Machine Row: 15, 12, 10*

Monday: Shoulders and Arms

1.) Barbell Seated Press: 20, 10, 8, 6, 4

2.) *Seated Lateral Raise: 15, 15, 12, 10*

3.) *Front Dumbbell Raise: 15, 15, 12, 10*

4.) Reverse Fly Machine: 15, 12, 10

5.) EZ Bar Standing Curl: 20, 10, 10, 8

6.) Close-Grip Barbell Bench Press: 20, 10, 10, 8

7.) *Incline Dumbbell Curls: 15, 12, 10*

8.) *One-Arm Overhead Dumbbell Extension: 15, 12, 10*

9.) *Concentration Curl: 15, 12, 10*

10.) *Cable Triceps Extension: 15, 12, 10*

Tuesday: Legs

1.) Standing Calf (toes in, toes out, parallel): 3 sets of 10 in each foot position, **30 TOTAL REPS EACH SET**

2.) Seated Calf: 3 sets of 10 in each foot position, **30 TOTAL REPS EACH SET**

3.) Calf Raise on Leg Press: 3 sets of 10 each foot position,

30 TOTAL REPS EACH SET

4.) Squat: 20, 15, 12, 10, 8, 6, 4

5.) Walking Lunge: 15, 10, 8, 6 (Each leg)

6.) Straight Leg Dead Lift: 20, 15, 10

7.) Lying Hamstring Curl: 20, 15, 10

8.) Quad Extension: 20, 15, 10

Wednesday: Chest and Back

1.) Barbell Incline Bench: 20, 10, 8, 6, 4

2.) Pull ups: 12, 10, 8, 6, 4

3.) Barbell Flat Bench: 10, 8, 6, 4

4.) Barbell Bent Over Row: 12, 10, 8, 6

5.) *Incline Dumbbell Flys: 15, 12, 10*

6.) *One-arm Dumbbell Row on Bench: 15, 12, 10*

7.) *Machine Fly: 15, 12, 10*

8.) *Seated Machine Row: 15, 12, 10*

Thursday: Shoulders and Arms

1.) Smith Seated Press: 20, 10, 8, 6, 4

2.) Barbell Shrug: 20, 15, 10, 8, 6

3.) Cable Side Raise: 15, 15, 12, 10

4.) Reverse Fly Machine: 15, 12, 12

5.) EZ Bar Standing Curl: 20, 10, 10, 8

6.) Cable Triceps Extension Palms Up and Palms Down:

20, 12, 10, 10 each position

7.) *Seated Dumbbell Curls: 15, 12, 10*

8.) *Two-Arm Overhead Barbell Extension: 15, 12, 10*

9.) *Concentration Curl: 15, 12, 10*

10.) *One-Arm Cable Triceps Extension: 15, 12, 10*

Friday: Legs

1.) Leg Press: 20, 15, 12, 10, 8, 6, 4

2.) Standing Lunge, barbell: 10, 10, 10, 10 (each leg)

3.) Front squat: 15, 10, 8, 6, 4

4.) Lying Hamstring: 15, 15, 10, 10

5.) Quad Extension: 15, 15, 10, 10

6.) Standing Calf (toes in, toes out, parallel): 3 sets of 10 in each foot position, **30 TOTAL REPS EACH SET**

7.) Seated Calf: 3 sets of 10 in each foot position, **30 TOTAL REPS EACH SET**

8.) Calf Raise on Leg Press: 3 sets of 10 in each foot position, **30 TOTAL REPS EACH SET**

Saturday: Off day

It is extremely effective if you stay true and really work 110%. It's all in your hands; no one will give you the results you want. You have to do it and work at it yourself. Become something the world has never seen - something extraordinary.

THE MASS MONSTER!

Example routine #4, after daily warm up

This example routine is for someone looking to put on muscle. It's a 6 week program designed in a specific way so we can work in as much volume as possible. This routine is a bit different than the first because there is no building phase. This should be done by an advanced lifter. I recommend doing routine #1 first if you are just getting started.

All 6 weeks of this program are the same. Stay true and consistent and good things will follow. Remember, we're looking for volume here. Pump the muscle with as much volume as we can in order to grow the muscle as much as possible.

It's critical to have a spotter/workout partner for this program. We are focused on lower reps in this routine, having someone to be able to spot you is crucial. Lift hard with intensity.

In this Become One program example:

- Train 6/7 days of the week, with one day off on Saturday
- Workouts are about 1 hour 30 minutes to 2 hours total including lift, warm up, and abs. This also depends on your focus level, so no talking or other funny business

- Workouts in italics are supersets (Do both together. For example if front and side raises are super setted, this means you do front raises first, then side raises upon finishing, without a break. Once both exercises have been completed, then rest. Then repeat for the designated number of sets.)
- 8 week program
- AMAP means "as many as possible"

Training split:

Monday: chest and biceps

Tuesday: back and triceps

Wednesday: legs

Thursday: shoulders

Friday: chest and back

Saturday: biceps and triceps

Monday: Chest and Biceps

1.) Flat Bench: 20, 15, 10, 8, 6, 4, 2 *(20 and 15 are meant to be a warm up since this is your first exercise)*

2.) Incline Bench: 10, 8, 6, 4

3.) Flat Cable Fly: 4 sets of 10

4.) High Cable Fly: 4 sets of 10

5.) Machine Chest Press: 12, 10, 8, 6

6.) *Arm Blaster Curl: 15, 10, 8, 6 (If you don't have access to an arm blaster, substitute with EZ bar curl)*

7.) *Single Arm Preacher: 4 sets of 10*

8.) Dumbbell Hammer Curl (alternating): 10, 10, 8, 6

Tuesday: Back and Triceps

1.) Lat Pull Down: 20, 15, 10, 10, 8, 6, 4 *(20 and 15 are meant to be a warm up since this is your first exercise)*

2.) T bar Row: 10, 10, 8, 8, 6

3.) Single Arm Dumbbell Row: 10, 10, 8, 8

4.) *Dumbbell Dead Lift: 10, 10, 8, 8*

   5) *Dumbbell Shrug: 4 sets of 20*

5.) Neutral Grip Pull Down: 4 sets of 10

6.) Dips Machine: 5 sets, 15, 12, 10, 8, 6

7.) EZ Bar Skull Crusher: 10, 10, 8, 6

8.) Dumbbell overhead: 10, 10, 8, 6

Wednesday: Legs

1.) Squat: 15, 12, 10, 8, 6, 4, 2

2.) Walking Lunge: 4 sets of 10 (each leg)

3.) Single Leg press on Leg Sled: 5 sets of 5

4.) Quad. Extension: 4 sets of 10

5.) Lying Hamstring Curl: 4 sets of 10

6.) Standing calf: 10, 10, 8, 8, 6

7.) Seated Calf: 10, 10, 8, 8, 6

Thursday: Shoulders

    1.) Seated Barbell Shoulder Press: 15, 12, 10, 8, 6, 4

    2.) Lateral dumbbell raise: 4 sets of 10

    3.) Dumbbell Front Raise (Alternating): 4 sets of 10

    4.) *Barbell Front Shrug: 15, 10, 8, 6*

    5.) *Barbell Rear Shrug: 15, 10, 8, 6*

    6.) Reverse Pec Deck: 4 sets of 10

Friday: Chest and Back

    1.) Incline Chest Press: 15, 12, 10, 8, 6, 4

    2.) Dumbbell Bench Press: 12, 10, 8, 6

    3.) Machine Fly: 4 sets of 10

    4.) Incline Fly: 4 sets of 10

    5.) Bent Over Barbell Row: 15, 12, 10, 8, 6

    6.) Seated Row: 4 sets of 10

    7.) Supinated Grip Lat Pull Down: 15, 12, 10, 8, 6

    8.) Upright Row: 4 sets of 10

Saturday: Arms

    1) Weighted Dips: 20, 15, 12, 10, 8, 6

    2) *Cable Press Down (overhand): 15, 12, 10, 8*

    3) *Cable press Down (underhand): 15, 12, 10, 8*

    4) Cable Overhead: 4 sets of 10

    5) Dumbbell Skull Crusher: 4 sets of 10

6) EZ Bar Curl: 15, 12, 10, 8, 6

7) Dumbbell Alternating Curl: 10, 8, 8, 6

8) *Standing Double Cable Curl: 4 sets of 10*

9) *Preacher Curl Machine: 4 sets of 10*

Sunday: Off day

As stated, each individual will respond differently to each workout. No two individuals are alike; each varies in weight, genetics, body type, etc. You must find what works best for your mind and body. This is crucial. Not everyone will have the same results, keep experimenting and your goals will come.

The Athlete

Example routine #5, after daily warm-up

This workout routine is for an athlete looking to get bigger, stronger, and faster. It's great for any type of athlete: football player, baseball player, basketball player, etc. It's split up so that you get the best of lifting to get bigger, but also supplemented with speed and agility to get faster! In any sport it's crucial to be as fastest as possible. So don't skip the speed days, they are critical to your success as an athlete.

In this Become One program example:

- Train 6/7 days of the week, with one day off on Sunday

- Workouts are about 1 hour 30 minutes depending on focus level, so no talking or funny business. You can get this done in 90 minutes if you work and go to the gym to do what you need to do.

- Workouts in italics are supersets (Do both together. For example if front and side raises are super setted, this means you do front raises first, then side raises upon finishing, without a break. Once both exercises have been completed, then rest. Then repeat for the designated number of sets.)

- 6 week program

- AMAP means "as many as possible"

Training split:

Monday: pushing (Chest, Shoulders, Triceps)

Tuesday: speed and agility

Wednesday: lower body

Thursday: speed and agility

Friday: pulling (Back and Biceps)

Saturday: speed and agility

Sunday: off day

Monday's Routine: Chest, shoulders, and triceps

1.) Bench Press: 20, 15, 10, 8, 6, 4, 4

2.) Incline dumbbell: 20, 15, 10, 8

3.) *Machine fly: 4 sets of 10*

4.) *Pushups: 4 sets of AMAP*

5.) Dumbbell shoulder press: 20, 15, 12, 10

6.) *Front raise: 10, 10, 10*

7.) *Side raise: 10, 10, 10*

8.) Dips: AMAP x 4 sets

9.) Dumbbell overhead: 20, 15, 10

Tuesday's Routine: Speed and agility

1. **Vertical jumps (Use vertical jump pole if possible to measure. If not, then use a wall or pole and mark measurements out)**

   - 5 jumps straight vertical

   - 5 jumps with a step

   - 5 jumps with weighted vest of vertical

   - 5 jumps with weighted vest with a step

2. **Mile run with weighted vest**

   - On treadmill or outside

3. **Water and 5 – 10 minute rest**

4. **Square cone drill (Sprint, side shuffle, back peddle, side shuffle. 4 cones in shape of a square, about 10-**

15 feet apart)

- 3 times one way, 3 times the other way

5. **Box jumps for HEIGHT**

   - 5 sets of 5 body weight

   - 5 sets of 5 with weighted vest

6. **Side shuffle drill (2 cones placed about 20 feet apart, side shuffle back and forth as many times as possible in 30 seconds)**

   - 5 sets

7. **Suicides to finish (Distance of each cone can vary, all up to the athlete)**

   - Complete 3 sets with bodyweight

   - Complete 3 sets with weighted vest

Wednesday's Routine: Lower Body

1.) Leg Press: 20, 15, 10, 8, 6, last set drop set

2.) Quad. Extension: 20, 15, 10, 20

3.) Lying Hamstring Curl: 20, 15, 10, 20

4.) *Step Ups (body weight or with dumbbells): 20, 15, 10*

**** If bodyweight is easy, then add dumbbells in order to increase the difficulty ****

5.) *Walking Lunges: 20, 15, 10*

6.) Single leg squat: 20, 15, 10, 20

7.) Standing calf raise: 3 sets x 10 reps each foot position

      (toes in, parallel, toes out…30 total reps each set)

8.) Seated calf raise: feet straight 3 sets x 20 reps

Thursday's Routine: Speed and agility

1. **Vertical jumps**

    - 5 jumps straight vert.

    - 5 jumps with a step

    - 5 jumps with weighted vest of vert.

    - 5 jumps with weighted vest with a step

2. **Sled push (40 yards, down and back)**

    - 5 sets, increasing weight each time

3. **Long jumps (Jump as far as you can each jump, go about 40 yards down and back)**

    - 2 sets bodyweight

    - 2 sets with weighted vest

4. **Water and 5 – 10 minute rest**

5. **Battle ropes (Hands alternate, up and down for 30 seconds)**

    - 5 sets, 30 seconds each set

6. **90 foot sprints**

    - 5 sprints

7. **Ladder drills (Go through 10 exercises, down and back through ladder)**

    - 3 sets

Friday's Routine: Start Back, then Bicep's

    1.) Pull ups: 4 sets x AMAP

    2.) Lat-Pull Down (palms toward your body, chin up): 20, 15, 12, 10

    3.) Neutral Grip Lat-Pull Down: 20, 15, 12, 10

    4.) One Arm Row on bench: 20, 15, 10

    5.) T- Bar Row: 20, 15, 12, 10

    6.) Dumbbell dead lift 20, 15, 12, 10

    7.) Straight bar curl: 20 x 4 sets

    8.) Preacher curl: 4 sets of 10

Saturday's Routine: Cardio

    1.) Mile run, no weighted vest

Sunday's Routine: Off day

*** It is very important to take off days and allowing your body to recover and heal. This is especially huge for a lifter who has just started to workout. Your body is not used to being under such stressful workouts, therefore it is vital to take rest. If you are sore, then there are many things you can do in order to reduce that. Stretching is a great way to help reduce soreness. Also, heat application, such as hot showers or soaking in a hot tub. Take today, rest up, and be ready to get back at it tomorrow. ***

The Creator

Example routine #6, after daily warm-up

I wanted to throw this one in here because it's a bit different, but for me is the most effective. Once you've established yourself in the gym and become more advanced, you're going to start to understand your body and it's weaknesses. Therefore you're not going to necessarily want a "specific" training plan because you're going to know what needs the most work. For example, I love to do what's called "instinctive training".

This means I'm not sure what exercises I'm going to perform when I go into the gym; I go by feel. So I know what I will be training (chest and biceps, or legs, or back, etc.), but I don't know what I will do when I step in the gym. Everything is based off of my experience and feel. After so many years of training and going through hundreds of different training plans, I know exactly what my body will respond to best and exactly what areas need the most attention. I lift like this most of the time that I lift because it allows me to really mix things up on an everyday basis. Therefore I only recommend doing this if you've been lifting for some time and know your body fairly well.

I won't give you a specific training split or exercises to perform, this one's on you. Once you've completed the workout plans and gained some experience, then you can create your own! Be creative, hit your weak points, and get to work.

"We're enslaved by the desire to be something that we're not instead of working towards something that we want to be."
-Cuong Quang

Part IV: The "education" to get there

"Most people say they want to look better, but not everyone is willing to do whatever it takes to achieve it."

-Taylor Haug

Action

Now comes the hardest step in the process: the action phase. I say this is the hardest because this is the step that takes the most effort, work, and time. This is the step that will make or break your results. You can create your vision, make your goals, and draw up a plan, but if you don't act on your dream, it will never happen - simple as that.

In this step we will be going over several things;
-   how to stay consistent

- how to have total commitment of your dream
- how to deal with injuries and setbacks
- how to prioritize your daily actions

You must take action; it's the only way to get the results you want. Don't sit back and wait for the results, take life by the horns and demand life to give you what's yours: your dream.

Notice the title says "education", not motivation. I like to call it education because motivation tends to not stick with people. An individual may get motivated for one day, then be lazy the next. But if the individual is "educated" on what he/she must do, they have a better chance of getting to their end result. Motivation is a temporary band-aid fix…but education is permanent information that will get you the help you need to make your dreams become a reality.

Consistency

The biggest component about your success in fitness is your consistency. Everyone can have a good day of working out or dieting. But it's doing it 365 days per year that brings the success you're looking for. You have to understand that all things in the universe operate on the same laws. This includes your success as an athlete. Newton's first law is that an object in motion will stay in motion, and an object at rest will remain at rest unless acted upon by an outside force. When an athlete starts to work out and sees quick results, generally they continue on because they see the results they want. Thus they continue to stay in motion! But as soon as they stop, all results will seize to come about. You must stay consistent every single day to see results. There is no other way to achieve your dreams.

If you look at successful people, they are creatures of habit. They are very deliberate about the things they do. They don't just do things when they want, they do things because they know the things they do will make them successful. It's a way of life. Being successful is a lifestyle not just an occurrence. They are successful everyday out of the habit of consistency, not luck and chance. They always want to win, they always want to work hard, and most importantly, they always want to get better. It's called consistency.

The difference between many unsuccessful people and successful people is that they are not consistent. Unsuccessful people only work hard when they feel like it. They wake up when they feel like it. They only get better when they feel like it. And some of them have never learned the concept of consistency. Champions and successful people are consistent everyday in what they do. Whether it's a disciplined sleep schedule, or a practice schedule, they do whatever they have to do every single day. They have a specific goal and vision in mind and their entire day is dedicated to that goal. No wasted opportunities. In everything you do you should be asking yourself, "how is this making me better?". In everything you do you should be asking yourself, "Am I going hard enough? Am I doing what it takes?" Everything you do in your day should help you get better…and most importantly, you should be consistent. Doing it every single day.

"Success whether you know it or not is very intentional and deliberate. There has never been a person that blew up and was successful and it happened by chance…"
- Eric Thomas

Successful people are not where they want to be because of chance and luck. They use their consistent hard work and effort to get themselves wherever they want to be in life. "I don't need luck because my hard work gets me where I want to be." So just remember, the next time you don't "feel like" working hard, there is somebody else out there getting better and one step closer to your dreams…

Shark Attack

Successful people are like the "sharks" of our world. Our world is filled with all sorts of people and living things, but there is just a small percentage of "sharks" in the world.

They're always on the prowl…looking for more. They're always looking for what they're going to eat next and what their next meal is going to be (meal or food = success). Not scared of anything around them and not afraid to challenge anyone. And they feed on your failure. When you fail and they get a taste of that "blood", there is nothing that can stop them from pouncing on you and taking your dreams away from you. Taking whatever they want from you because all they want is success. Once they taste that "blood", they're on the lookout so they can snatch and take what's rightfully theirs…
THEIR PREY!

-Taylor Haug

This is how you must be if you want to be successful. If you want to be the best then you have to be willing to take on any challenge and take what's yours. You have to be a go-getter. A shark doesn't sit around and wait for their food. They go and take it. Your dreams aren't going to magically appear and come to you. You have to go take what you think you deserve. And let me tell you something, it's going to be hard at first. But when you taste that "blood" or success for the first time, there's no going back. Once you taste that success for the first time, you will continue to want more and more and before you know it, you will be one of those creatures. One of the few "sharks" of the world. Not afraid of anything and feasting off of others failure….taking what's yours.

Total commitment

Everyone has dreams and aspirations. However most people will fail and never reach them because of one thing: lack of total commitment. People will fail not because they don't have the skill or talent, but because they're not willing to give 100% to their cause. Most people aren't willing to make sacrifices and lay it all on the line for what they want and believe in.

"At any moment, you have to be willing to sacrifice what you are, for what you will become."
- Eric Thomas

If you want to achieve greatness, then you have to have total commitment of the mind body and spirit. And this is going to include sacrificing things in life. Sacrificing who you are now, for what you will become in the future. Whether it's skipping out on hanging out with your friends, working an extra job, etc., you have to do whatever it takes to reach your dreams and goals. Total commitment = 100%. If you're going to give 99%, then you might as well throw in the towel. Because somewhere out there, there is someone working 100% that is going to take your dream from you.

Burned out…

"If you guys are really wondering if you are burned out mentally….then take a day off and go to your local hospital. Go to the cancer wing and look at a 4 year old who won't ever see their teenage years, let alone their next birthday. Go and see a mentally or physically retarded. Go and see a soldier who just came back from war who doesn't have a leg anymore. Stare that guy down. Look at him in his eyes and tell him, as you stand there with 2 perfectly capable legs, that you are 'burned out'. Tell him that you don't want to use them anymore. See if that doesn't kill him right then and there. Because he would do anything to have that opportunity."

-*Greg Plitt (Actor, model, US Army)*

Stop making excuses for yourself. Stop telling yourself that it's too hard and you can't keep moving. Stop telling yourself that you don't have what it takes to accomplish the task at hand. Because somewhere out there, there is someone who has it worse than you. There will always be someone who wants to be where you are. So don't take what you have for granted. Take what you have and use it to be the best you can be and don't complain about what you don't have! Why fail when success is an option? Don't stop because you're feeling a little "burned out" Keeping working until you make your dreams come into reality. Before you know it, you will be on top of the mountain…looking down on your "competition".

Lift 100% or don't lift at all

Why go to the gym and not give it your all day in and day out? In my personal opinion, too many people go to the gym without a purpose and sense of urgency. The reason we go to the gym is to achieve results and become better versions of ourselves. But the only way to do that is to lift 100% every single day. Going to the gym without a purpose is just a waste of time and money, simple as that. 100% commitment to a single goal is how results are achieved. Without full commitment, results are complacent or non-existent.

I understand lifting for some is not as serious as it is for others. But I think regardless of one's goals when going to the gym, each individual should still give total commitment to the task at hand. If your goal is to lose weight, go 100%. If your goal is gain muscle, go 100%. Even if you have smaller goals like achieving wash board abs, or benching a certain amount of weight, you still must go 100% to achieve the fastest results.

There is no texting or taking pictures or any funny business. Just do what you need to do to become the best. There is a time and place for taking pictures of yourself, but mid workout isn't the place. There is a time and place for answering text messages, but during your workout isn't that time. Do what you need to do with no distractions and focus in on the task at hand! Lift 100% or don't lift at all.

What's the fastest path from point A to point B? A straight line of course. But what's faster? Walking the straight line? Or sprinting it? The choice is up to you.

So if you're really serious about achieving your dreams, think about how much you're putting in. Think about your commitment. Think about your actions at the gym. Because if you're not putting in 100%, you can kiss your dreams goodbye.

Winning and losing

Losing is a very important part of being a athlete. Everyone will lose at some point or another. Everyone will lose. The difference between champions and losers is how the champions take losing. They hate losing more than they like winning. If they lose, you can bet that they are going to lose sleep over it. You can bet that they are going to take that loss to heart. And you can bet that they are going to do whatever it takes to not lose again! So why are average people okay with losing? Why are they okay with the way they look? Average people have to be so sick and tired of settling for who are currently are that they change from average to extraordinary. Don't be okay with the results you continue to receive. Don't be okay with "mediocrity". Do whatever it takes to win and be the best looking person on the planet. The difference between most people and myself is that I am obsessed with becoming the best on the planet. I continue to look at myself in the mirror and want to be better every single day. Therefore every time I step in the gym, I am fully committed to becoming something great and you can do this too.

All athletes lose at some point in their career. Even when they believe they are in tip top shape, they still lose that's just the nature of winning and losing. But I believe that losing shows a true reflection of who you really are. It reflects on how you prepared for that contest or show. How did you train? Were you in the gym every day doing what it takes to be a champion? Were you making sacrifices to miss out on some fun time with your friends? How you compete at that contest will completely reflect on your training. Now I'm not saying that if you trained your heart out, that you are going to win every show…but if you train your heart out, I can tell you that, no matter what, you will give the other guys a run for their money and you will leave that contest with your head held high because you know you did whatever it took to win. But this doesn't just pertain to people who compete, this is for everyone who wants to lose weight or gain muscle for themselves. Every single time you step on that scale it should be the same feeling. You should feel as if you are competing every time you step on that scale if you really want to be the best. Have you been doing all you can to reach your dream? Every day is one step closer…

So the choice is up to you, continue to be satisfied or be the best the world has ever seen.

"It's not all about winning, but why train for second place?"
Sensei Scott Haug, 6th Degree Black Belt in Isshin Ryu Karate, Kyokushin Karate Knockdown Champion

Priorities

If you want to be successful then you have to understand what is important tp you and what is not. You have to have your priorities in check each and every day in order to progress. Too many people do not have their priorities straight when it comes to achieving something. They never get far because they are easily distracted by things in life. Everything you do you should put into a "category":

- Emergency

- very important

- Important

- kind of important

- not important

Everything you do throughout your day should go through this checklist; from top to bottom. Everyone's activities will be placed differently throughout this list. But the reason why people fail in fitness is because they do not place it ahead of other things in life. If you truly want results then sacrifices must be made.

I will give you some examples. For me, saying no was never a problem. My friends understood how important my personal health and fitness was growing up. They understood that at certain times, I had to finish up my priorities. I wouldn't always "skip" out on my friends; I just might show up a little later than everyone else. What I'm trying to say is that missing an hour of your friends "play time" isn't going to kill you. Missing one party on a weekend doesn't mean they won't be there partying again soon. Know what is important to you and you will start to make progress in the right direction. You will not lose friends by saying no….let me repeat myself, you will not lose friends because you say no. If you lose "friends" for saying no to partying on a weekend, let it be clear that they probably weren't your friends anyways.

Losing weight and gaining muscle isn't an easy task, let alone dedicating yourself to the training you must go through to get there. However, if you know what's important to you then it will make your task that much easier. You will find yourself more prepared, more ready for what's ahead.

I will give you something you can relate to. Have you ever gone into a test at school like, "oh yeah baby I'm ready for this, let's do this. Give me the test already because I'm going to ace this! It's a great feeling knowing you're ready and going to succeed. And then there's the other side, going into a test knowing you're going to fail. Maybe you stayed up late the night before or maybe decided to hang out with your girl or your friends instead of studying, knowing you should have prepared more so you had a better chance on that exam.

How is this different from your fitness goals? Walking into a gym with your head held high knowing that you're losing weight or gaining muscle every time you set foot in the gym is an unbelievable feeling. It's not being cocky. It's being confident in yourself that you know your becoming something great. Think about your training. Most of you train for a couple weeks then quit; you aren't training. You say you train but you don't really train. Going to the gym twice a week isn't training. Dieting for a week isn't training. Going to the gym and socializing isn't training. If you want be the best the world has ever seen, then you have to be at the grind every single day - lifting, dieting, cardio, etc. Having that "first one in last one out" mentality. You have to prepare yourself for the task that's ahead, preparing your mind body and spirit for the war that's about to happen. And the way to do this is to have your priorities in order. Know what is important to you. Don't be afraid to say no and take the difficult road. Work and be the greatest the world has ever seen.

Setbacks

Setbacks inevitably happen to every athlete at one time or another. No matter what the athlete does, setbacks will happen, whether it's an injury, sickness, etc. However, the goal is to not get setback frequently. In the Become One program, our aim is to train as long as we can without suffering an injury. We want to work out in a healthy way because we cannot accomplish our goals and dreams if were sitting on the sidelines plagued by injury. I take pride in staying as healthy as I possibly can. I hear all the time from athletes, "my leg bothers me, I think I pulled a muscle", etc. I have athletes that tell me something different bothers them every week! Work out in a healthy way, and we'll be able to reach your goals and dreams faster.

"Every setback is a setup for a comeback" Every set back has significance. However, how you handle the set back is most important. You have to realize why it's happening to you. At the time you could think it's the most miserable thing in the world. But what you don't realize is that the set back actually allows you to come back stronger than ever and here's why.

When you have that set back you regain that drive and that itch to get back to whatever it is you're missing. You're so fed up with the fact you can't do what you love. But this whole process is just preparing your mind for the return. I know when I have a setback and can't workout for a long period of time, I am like a lion in a cage; I just want to get out! I start to regain that itch where I know once I can lift again I'm going to lift harder than ever before. (But if you're like me this is you every time you set foot in a gym, we don't wait for setbacks)

Having a setback gives you a new foundation. Every person's body needs a rest at some point or another. Giving yourself a rest is a great way to start fresh. Many people are too stubborn to give their bodies a rest for fear of losing days to train. However, rest needs to be taken whether an athlete likes it or not. A setback can give you just that - a fresh new start.

Setbacks aren't always what you'd expect them to be. Take them with positivity and good things will result. Take them with negativity however, and they will hinder your performance and health. Continue to look at the larger vision at hand and without a doubt a setback can absolutely help you.

If it was easy, everyone would do it

A lot of people complain. They complain about where they are in life. They complain about their training or the grind. They complain about what they have. They complain about every little thing in life, thinking that complaining is going to make a miracle happen. But here's the reality of life: if it was easy everyone would do it.

If you want to be average then go ahead and complain. Because the only thing complaining brings you is wasted time. While you're complaining: there's someone out there getting better, making more money than you, and turning their average life into a dream life. And here's the thing about complaining, it's not a redeemable value. While you're complaining about whatever it is you're complaining about, you're eating away at the time you could be using to get better. No wasted opportunities. Every moment of the day you should be asking yourself, "what could I be doing to make myself better?" Stop complaining and make your dream happen because it's not going to just show up one day. Your dream is created by the work you finish every day. Lay the "brick" down every day to build that "mansion" you have been dreaming about. Instead of complaining, start appreciating everything that comes your way. The little things that may go wrong may show you a new, improved path. The biggest lessons in life come from winning and losing. And right when the thing you complain about is taken away, you wish it were here - for example your job, a certain person, etc.

If it was easy everyone would do it. Everyone would be rich. Everyone would be a pro athlete. Everyone would have their dream job. So how do these select few accomplish their dreams and aspirations? No wasted opportunities. They understand that they have to do more than every other person in the world to be the best. There are 24 hours in a day. Successful people make use of every hour in the day. They get up earlier than the rest of society. They stay up later. They do whatever it takes to make their dream become a reality. It's not easy to make sacrifices. It's not easy to do this on an daily basis. But hence the title: if it was easy, everyone would do it.

Our bodies are free, thus the vast majority of people take them for granted! We don't have to pay a "body tax" each year so people can easily do what they want with them. It takes a very different person in this world to take care of their bodies in a positive manner. But let's put it in this perspective: we keep our bodies for 80 years, on average. Why not have one you can be proud of. Why not have a body that will help you last longer than those average 80 years. It's not easy…but if it was then everyone would be in perfect shape. Take the harder route because the person you become in the process is more important than the result.

Who cares what people think

No matter what you choose to do in life, there will always be people who try to bring you down. There will always be "haters" and critics who like to question everything you do. But it's important to stay focused and focus on you. No one is going to see your vision or your dream. Not everyone is going to support what you do. But you cannot let these people make you deviate from your goals and dreams.

In all walks of life there are people who criticize everything and everyone. Whether its sports, politics, at your job, etc., people will always question the greats. Everyone is different, which means not everyone will understand what it is you must do. Only you know what you must do…no one else can tell you that. If you know deep down within that something is right for you, then go for it. Don't let the outside world tell you how to live your life. Stay focused on where you want to go and what you must do.

One example I can give you is with the goal card I spoke of earlier in the goals section of this book. I personally keep a goal card taped to the back of my phone, and almost daily I am questioned about what it stands for. Numerous people see my phone and question me about what it is I have taped to the back of my phone. I tell them what it stands for, and almost 100% of people look at me like I have three heads after I tell them. They question why I do it, and/or whether it works or not. However, I disregard all comments because I know what works for me. Regardless of whether they think what I do is right doesn't matter to me. Like Emerson once said, "To be great is to be misunderstood." If you want to be great, you must go against what most people believe is right. Stay focused on you and what you plan to accomplish.

Control what you can control. Simple as that. There is no telling what others will say or do, but that's not in your jurisdiction. Your focus is on your goals and dreams and no one else's. Your job isn't to live out another's dream and vice versa, you must do what God put you on this earth to do and only you know what that is. But don't let others tell you what you can and cannot do. Reach deep down and fulfill your own destiny and I promise you will be successful at whatever it is you must do.

Time

I hear it every single day from people "I don't have enough time to work out…". Stop right there. Every person in this world has enough time in the day to do whatever it is they need to do. There is always time in the day to do the things you're committed to. The reason why many people say there is not enough time is because of their commitment level. When someone is committed it doesn't matter how busy their day is, they will make time for the gym. They will make time for their workout. For me, I will go to the gym at 2 am if I have to if that's what it takes for me to get my lift in for the day. That's because I'm committed to becoming something great. I will not take "no time" for an answer.

How can an individual replace the "no time" mindset? Not better time management, but better activity management. It means becoming more effective by starting this program and saying yes to the things that will make you successful and no to everything else. It means being obsessed with the end result and making sure nothing gets in the way in the pursuit to get there. It means changing habits, replacing old complacent ones with ones that will help you grow. And lastly, it means gaining the champion mindset to make sure you become number one in whatever your field is.

Often times it's about replacing actions that aren't productive with ones that are, such as working out and exercising. If an individual looks at his/her day, there are more things than we realize that we can do better to be more productive. Something as simple as, instead of listening to music to and from work, you listen to a motivational tape to boost your positive energy levels for the day. This sounds minuscule, but this is what you may need in order to get your butt to the gym every day. Maybe instead of hanging around with your friends three times a week, you hang out twice and hit the gym one extra day. These are little things, but if you truly want to accomplish your goals they must be done. In the world of working out, it's the little things that make you great. It's not all about what happens in the gym. Often times what happens outside the gym takes precedence over your actual workout.

What to listen to when working out

This is a subject that often gets over looked. To some it may seem pretty simple and straight forward. However, this is a topic that I have experimented with for some time now and have found that what goes into my headphones often controls my workout. I have tried many things over the years - music, instrumentals, audio books, motivation, no music, absolute silence, the whole nine yards. To my surprise, each one of these that I have tried definitely made an impact on my lift.

For example, I experimented with silence or no music for a while in an attempt to put all my focus on the task at hand. I tried to focus all of my power on the contraction of the muscles so that my mind didn't wander on anything else. This definitely helped, but only to a certain degree. For me, what silence lacked was rhythm. I like to keep the same rhythm throughout as I lift. But I still go back to this method when I need to refocus my mind on the task. This is a great way to learn how to contract each muscle in your body as there are no distractions.

Looking at music, I have tried all genres. But for me music is a big downfall and I'll tell you why. For most people, they like to pick music that gets them really pumped up. Maybe one may choose heavy metal or aggressive rap in order to increase their intensity level. However, the problem with this is what I like to call "the roller coaster workout". Where you're first big exercise may be great, but your second may be not so good. And your four exercises may be fantastic, but your fifth lacks energy.

For instance, let's look at an average chest day. Usually an individual will start with bench press and typically go quite heavy. So therefore they pick a song to get them very amped and excited. They crush the bench press, and then move on to incline. However, as the workout progresses, they lose energy and motivation to keep going because they expended it all on the first exercise. So they scramble to find another song to get themselves to peak again. Because of this "roller coaster" theory, the secondary exercises do not receive the same attention and energy that your primary ones do.

To try and eliminate this I took a unique approach. I tried only instrumental music for a couple of weeks. This would help to keep my at the same level for the entire time I was at the gym, not too high but not too low. This would also help to keep my rhythm for the duration of my routine. To my astonishment this did help my workouts no question. Whether it was 10 minutes in or 90 minutes in, I was able to give out the same attention and energy to each exercise that I performed. This works for me, it may not work for everyone but I would definitely recommend it for someone having trouble with energy levels and the "roller coaster workout".

Another type is motivation such as videos are a great way to stay motivated during your workout. I especially enjoy listening to such videos while warming up in order to get my mind ready for the task at hand. It allows me to stay focused and drain out all other the things that are irrelevant to my workout. Websites such as You Tube have hundreds of videos and motivation channels to choose from. Pick a couple and get working.

As stated, everyone is different. Maybe you may not experience the "roller coaster workout" as I like to call it. But it's crucial to understand what works best for you that will allow you to perform the best workout you possibly can. Experiment with what you can, and then choose the audio that will make you unstoppable.

Be creative

In order to make the best gains you possibly can, you must be creative with your workout plans. It's not enough to just go in the gym and do the same thing every time. Your body will eventually adjust and therefore minimize, if not stop, your gains. Therefore you must experiment and try new things in order to get your desired end result.

Take what Arnold Schwarzenegger called the "shocking principle" for example:

"When we were training for bodybuilding competitions, shocking meant doing things like stripping – starting at the heavy end of the dumbbell rack and doing six reps of overhead press with 100 pound dumbbells, and then without resting, lift

the 90 pound dumbbells, then the 80, 70, 60, 50, 40. Back then, lifting 40 pounds was a piece of cake. But with the shock of dropping from each weight with no rest, 40 pounds felt like 110. Afterward, I couldn't even move my arms without pain. But the muscles grew, because I had given them the shock they so desperately wanted.

One of my favorite shocking methods was to go outside with 250 pounds on a barbell and a training partner. Our bodies were so used to doing 10 sets of squats that we could do it asleep. So I did 20 reps, and passed the barbell to my training partner, who lifted it into the squat position and did 20 reps. Without setting the bar down, he passed it back to me, and I did 20 reps again. Or maybe I could only do 19. We went on and on like this, never letting the bar touch the ground, until we could barely move. But again, the muscles grew, because we'd broken up the tedium of doing 10 sets of squats inside.

Those shocks are obviously major ones. For you right now, shocking might mean that when you go for a 15 minute walk, you spend a few of the minutes moving as fast as you can. Maybe you've worked up to jogging. When you go for a daily jog, sprint as hard as you possibly can a few times.

Switch it up. Think consciously about shocking your system with something that it hasn't adapted to yet.

Keep moving forward toward the healthiest version of

yourself, and don't let your muscles get bored."

This is one way to get creative and keep your muscles moving in ways they aren't used to. Another method is starting with weak points on your body with each lift. For instance if today is leg day, instead of starting with quads switch it up and start with calves. For me, calves have always lagged behind other leg muscles like my quads and hamstrings. Therefore starting with calves will allow me to focus first on my weak point then hit my strong points later. Another example might be with shoulders. Instead of starting with a general pressing movement, why not start with rear delts first. Often times our front delts get lots of work because they get worked with other muscle groups, when maybe our rear delts lag behind. Therefore starting with rear delts will allow you to address the weak point first and "shock" the muscle.

Training partners

Another way to be creative with your workouts is to add a workout partner. Often times when people workout by themselves they get lazy and lay back because no one is there to push them or keep them accountable. Having a workout partner can really turn things around because it will help you get the next level of training that you need to reach your goals. However, if you are not disciplined about who you choose to workout with, it can become a social hour rather than a workout session. It is crucial that you find someone who is as serious as you about reaching their goals as you are. If you fail to do this, your workouts will become worse than they were before.

Working out with another person is like two warriors going to battle: there is a code of honor. It sounds crazy but it's quite true. I workout with a partner because I know when I feel like passing out, he/she is there to catch me and keep me on my feet. When he/she is ready to quit, I am there to give them the extra energy needed to do another set. If my partner hits 225 lb on bench, then I have to because there is no way he can beat me. It's a win/win when you find that right person for the role. But make no mistake you have to find the right one. A workout partner should be a catalyst for your workout, not a cancer.

If you'd like to see two individuals work together to accomplish something remarkable, take a look at 8x Mr. Olympia champion Dorian Yates training videos. Now obviously you and your workout partner do not have to be as intense, but the overall goal should be the same. The overall goal should be to help one another achieve the goals you set out to accomplish and to become something extraordinary. Find the workout partner that will push you past your limits and keep you accountable, then watch your workouts go to the next level.

Leave your own legacy

I encourage you to leave your own mark on this Earth. I want to see everyone succeed and leave their own legacy behind. But you can't do that wanting to be someone else. Be inspired to leave something that this world has never seen. Think about that for a moment…there can only be one you - no one is identical to you. Therefore you are special…you have something inside of you that no one can match. You can leave something extraordinary that only you can do. Never be in pursuit of something that isn't yours. There can be only one Arnold Schwarzenegger, there can only be one Taylor Haug, and there can only be one of you. Be in pursuit of your own legacy, and leave something that's special.

I hear a lot of people say "I want to look like him!" or "I want to have abs like that celebrity does!" I encourage you to stop looking at others and create your own greatness. Know within yourself that you can look better. You can create something even better than what other people have because it's unique to you! Of course, as stated earlier in this book, others can be used as inspiration to help you get to another level. But strive to be better. Don't settle for something that someone else has already created, be something unique.

What does achieving greatness mean to you? Something that people must realize is that the definition of success is different for everyone. Depending on your job, dream, role, etc., success will be different for each individual. Nobody has the life you do. Nobody had the same childhood that you did. Nobody has the same skills, traits, or genetics you do. You're different and unique. You have something within you that you can offer the world that nobody has ever seen before. It's crucial that you know this.

Nobody will ever be Michael Jordan. He was unique, and no matter how much people want to compare others to him, MJ left his own mark on the game of basketball. Lebron James doesn't want to be like MJ, he wants to be better. He wants to leave his own mark and legacy on the game of basketball. Now I'm not trying to go into a heated debate but it's quite true.

You are you. Strive to be the best you can be, not be like someone else. Leave a mark that's only yours. Leave that unique mark that says I'm here. It's time to do something that the world has never seen before…it's your time.

Rack your weights

This is something that rarely gets done anymore. And the reason why I include this topic in this book is because it needs to be done every single workout. We go to the gym to get in top physical shape, which means we lift weights. It's part of the workout to put your weights on the bar and to unload them off! It's part of the workout to lift the dumbbells off the rack and to put them back on. Unless you're Mr. Olympia champion Ronnie Coleman, there is no reason why you should not put back your weights.

If you are strong enough to use them, then you are strong enough to put them back. I have seen women and elderly people not able to use certain equipment because people fail to put their weights back. A 45lb plate may be light for some people, but to others it's heavy. Sometimes it's so heavy that they can't use the equipment because they can't re-rack the weights that were used before them.

It is common courtesy for all, and that's all anyone asks for. Treat people's belongings with respect, just as if they are in your house treating your belongings with respect. Put your weights back and be respectful to everyone. It will make you all the better for it.

Tracking your workouts

I have found that tracking your workouts can be useful in order to see your progress. Many people look into the mirror to try and see results. But many times the changes won't come right away, especially to the eyes that see your body every day. It can be very discouraging to not see physical changes for some time. But this is where tracking your workouts comes into play.

If you track your workouts you will be able to see just how much you are improving because the numbers don't lie. You will be able to notice strength gains in your numbers before you will be able to notice changes in your physical appearance. This will keep you on track and keep you in a positive state of mind while trying to reach your goals.

A big positive to tracking your workouts is adding/dropping exercises that aren't working for you. If you're doing squats for example and notice you haven't been able to increase your weight or rep range for four weeks, then maybe it's time to switch it up and go with something else to help you get over that plateau. If you didn't write these things down, this may be something you wouldn't notice. It's the little things that count, if you can catch something early on you're bound to reach your goals faster.

How do I track my workouts? There are a variety of ways to do this:
- small notebook
- phone apps

- Microsoft excel spreadsheet
- Workout specific journal (bodybuilding.com sells these)

Each of these has their own positives and negatives; you just have to find what's easiest for you.

I understand that this may be time consuming during your workout, but this will make a difference if you are struggling. What I stated before is a great example. Seeing those strength gains in your numbers is the best way to stay motivated along your journey. It isn't always about what you look like. As long as you keep progressing in the right direction everything will come together.

Another benefit is to see which workout routines work best for you. Every workout you do will show different gains for your body. Writing down those gains will allow you to see which regimen works best for you. I know if I go back to my old workout journals I will be able to see which workout routine worked best for me. Therefore if I am looking to mix things up, I can go back and choose the one that gave me the best results instead of wondering what helped me and what didn't. We've already done our trial and error, we don't want to go through that again if we don't have too.

Keep moving forward; take the journey step by step. Your dream isn't going to come all at once. Be patient, and with each step taken, you will become a better version of yourself.

Taking progress pictures

Taking progress pictures can be a great way to measure how you're doing and give yourself a little extra "education" to get you to where you want to be. No matter where you are on your fitness journey, you can take pictures today. You can take pictures now so that in a month's time, for example, you can take more pictures and see how you're doing. Some questions you can ask yourself are:

- Is my workout program doing myself a justice?
- Do I need to change my workout plan?
- What weak points do I need to address?
- Am I working hard enough?
- (to answer the question above) Do I need a workout partner to push me further?

Everyone works out for different reasons. For bodybuilders, it isn't about how much weight you lift, but rather how you look. They are concerned more with proportion, symmetry, and size. But for power lifters, they are on the other side of the spectrum. Rather than their look, they want to increase their weights as much as they can. Therefore progress pictures may not be as beneficial to them. For the recreational lifter, progress pictures can definitely be utilized.

Time frames for these photos have to be separated by good amounts of time, however. If I take pictures on Monday, and then again on the following Saturday I can't expect to see a difference. The time frame must be fairly realistic. I recommend doing an 8 week period for your progress pictures. If you really push yourself, you will see progress.

Lots of people who aim to better themselves jump into weight lifting but have no sense of direction. They will lift for a couple of months then finally come to the conclusion, "what am I truly doing here?". If you are to truly master your body, you must be able to gauge how far you've come. It's easy to tell people you lift and feel healthier. But do you look healthier? Taking progress pictures allows you to finally be able to see your hard work paying off. And if you don't see progress, then maybe it's the kick in the butt you need to push yourself that much farther.

How to take these pictures:

You can either take these yourself, or have someone take them for you (which I recommend because it's much easier). Obviously for our purposes we don't need a highly sophisticated camera, your phone camera will do just fine. Taking these pictures may be different for everyone depending on your goals. But it's easy to start with simple pictures to monitor your progress. Please note, these pictures are for you. Therefore you shouldn't be discouraged to take these. They will only help you better yourself.

To start, you can take four basic photos as follows: Just completely relax, do not flex any muscle while taking these four.

    1.) relaxed front

    2.) relaxed right side

    3.) relaxed back

    4.) relaxed left side

Keep these in your archive and then take more after 8 weeks to measure progress!

Now if you're an aspiring bodybuilder or physique competitor, then you can take slightly more advanced photos. For a bodybuilder, they must hit several different poses while on stage to show off their bodies. These are the main 8:

    1.) Front Double Biceps

    2.) Front Lat Spread

    3.) Side Chest

    4.) Side Triceps

5.) Back Double Biceps

6.) Back Lat Spread

7.) Abdominal & Thigh

8.) Most muscular

Take a photo for each pose in addition to the basic four. This will give you a complete overview of your body and how it looks before your start your training regime.

Be wise about choosing a personal trainer.....

Now I have to put this in here because it needs to be addressed. Good personal training these days can be very hard to find. Is there good personal training out there? Of course there is! But you have to look hard to find it.

In today's world it's very easy to get taken up by a "wanna be" personal trainer that has no idea what they are doing. I've lifted at lots of gyms around the country and can say from personal experience that about 50% of people that I see "certified" should not be teaching anyone about working out. They are either not healthy themselves or are teaching from a book! It's very easy to just go online and get certified to be a personal trainer without any experience.

Personal training should be done from experience. I

have never made anyone do anything that I have never done before. Why would I? I would never make one of my clients do a workout or exercise that I have never tested on myself. Why? Because I want to make sure my clients to the exercise right and to make sure that the workout/exercise is beneficial to my client! I don't want my client to not have results, so I must make sure that what I give them works.

Personal training is a profession, but it should also be a passion. I stated this earlier in the book and I'll state it again. My job as a personal trainer is not to take money from my clients and then walk away. My job is to guarantee your results and to stay with you every step of the way. This means helping you both in the gym and outside the gym. As a personal trainer, I will give you everything you need to be successful: the tools, the mindset, the plan, the accountability, etc. My job is to give you everything you would like to have, and then some, so that in the future you don't need my help anymore. I will give you the results you want and if I don't you get your money back…

Why am I telling you this? So that you know what to look for in a trainer when and if you seek one out.

How do I make sure that he/she is a good personal trainer?

You can ask them questions:

- What's your workout experience?

- How many years have you been training/working out?

- How many clients have you trained?

- What are your clients success rate?

- What are your accomplishments in this specific field? (Power lifting, bodybuilding, etc.)

- Where did you receive your certification?

This may seem silly, but I know if I was giving my money to someone I would want to make sure they are perfect for the job. So before you go out and about just choosing any trainer, make sure they are the perfect fit for you. Find that person that will push you to the limit and make you the best they possibly can.

Closing statement

"It's a wondrous thing, that a decision to act releases energy in the personality. For days on end a person may drift along without much energy. Having no particular sense of direction and having no will to change. Then, something happens to alter the pattern. It may be something very simple and inconsequential in itself. But it stabs awake, it alarms, it disturbs. In a flash, one gets a vivid picture of oneself, and it passes. The result is decision. Sharp, definitive decision. In the wake of the decision, yes, even as a part of the decision itself, energy is released. The act of decision sweeps all before it, and the life of the individual maybe changed forever."

- Howard Thurman

You now have all the tools you need to become something great. Now it's on you…

You can teach someone exactly what they need to do to become something special. But what you can't teach is the "want" to get there. You can't teach someone to want to become something more; that must come from within. No one will be on your back telling you when to go to the gym, what to eat, and what you need to work on. You must find it within yourself; the intrinsic motivation to become something the world has never seen before.

Remember this: there is nothing wrong with the system. In today's society, people try to short cut the success. There will always be a new pill that "helps you lose weight faster". There will always be the new ab machine you see on the infomercials that "guarantees the 6 pack". And of course you will see the people on the magazines who say you can shortcut your way to a better body. All of these shields the truth! There is no shortcut to success. You must put in the hours of work to look the best you possibly can. No "pill" or "secret machine" can do that for you. There is no substitute for hard work. There is nothing wrong with the system, it has worked for years. The only reason why people come up with these new things is to try and cheat the system or to sell you their product to make money. Work hard and work hard again, there is no other way.

You are a creator, create what you'd like to become.
-Taylor Haug

Everyone has something within themselves that they can show the world. No two people will ever look exactly alike! So why not take it upon yourself to give the world another masterpiece they can admire? You only receive one body; why not make it the best it can possibly be?

I would like to commend you for finishing this journey with me. But it doesn't stop here. Keep pressing forward! The journey within yourself will never end, always remember that. It's an ongoing journey that will be with you forever. If you ever need the encouragement to continue on, I will be right around the corner. Just crack open the book and I will be ready to help.

Become One with who you were meant to be!

Special thanks

I would like give a special thanks to my parents, Scott and Sandy, for believing in me in everything that I do. It's a wondrous thing knowing that you have my back no matter what it is I try to pursue. Without your help, love, and support, none of this would have been possible. You're my parents, but better yet, you're my teachers. Thank you for showing me the way towards success and greatness. Love you guys forever and always! To my mom, you are the strongest woman I know. You have taught me that anything is possible with the heart to get there. You have changed my life with just the little things you do, day in and day out. Thank you, and nothing you do goes unnoticed. I love ya! To my dad, you are my hero and always will be. You're superman to me. You put your heart and soul into everything you do and showed me that anything is possible. We'll always be partners in crime, and I thank you for everything you do for me. I love ya!

I would like to give a special thanks to my brother, Scott Jr, who has shown me what it takes to be the best. You are the hardest worker I know and you are a true testament to a success story. I appreciate all your help and support. You bring me to a higher level everyday and I appreciate you pushing me to go farther than I ever thought I could. I could not have done all of this without you at my side, thank you for everything. Love you bro! See you at the top.

I would like to thank my sister and brother in-law, Beth and Jason, for creating awesome memories with me. I am thankful for your support and couldn't ask for a better sister and brother to have in my life. Love you guys! Love you Blakley!

I would like to thank my extended family for always supporting me. My wonderful grandmother Francis, you always give love to everyone and always seem to bring a smile to everyone's face. To my nanna and grandfather, Kathie and Glenn, thank you for your wisdom and love along my journey in life. Thank you for always providing me with your love and support. My Uncle Jon and cousins Jonathan, Matt, and Nick, you guys always provide me the support and help I need. Thank you for your love and support. Love all you guys!

I would like to thank my partner in crime and my best

friend Cuong Quang. You have come such a long way and have taught me so much along your journey. I appreciate everything you have done for me, it never goes unnoticed. But the grind and journey never stops, keep pressing forward. I know you will be one of the greats someday, and I will be here with you every step of the way. Thank you my friend, see you at the top.

I would like to thank my beautiful girlfriend Sarah. You are there for me no matter what and I thank you for that. You make me so happy, and you make my face hurt daily from all of the smiling and laughing we do together. You work so hard at your goals in life, and you inspire me to dream bigger and work harder every single day. Thanks for being behind me no matter what path I pursue in life. I love you, and can't wait to see what we accomplish together.

I would like to give a special thanks to the Reynolds family for taking me in and treating me like part of the family. You guys showed me that it's not always about the things you have, but rather the people that you surround yourself with. The entire duration of my stay with you guys was nothing but loving, caring, and of course fun. To Mr. and Mrs. Reynolds, I thank you for treating me like a son. It is a debt that I can never fully repay, so I thank you guys for that. To Tucker, Dakota, Cordell, and Dalton, I love you guys and you will always be family to me!

I would like to thank the rest of my friends: Brendon, Kevin, Steve, James, Robert, Ja'quan, T.J, Brandon, Winfred, Mike, and Dalton. I apologize if I forgot anyone! Thank you guys for sharing incredible memories with me. All the love and support goes a long way and it never goes unnoticed. I love you guys! I have the greatest friends in the world and I couldn't ask for more from you guys. Thanks for dealing with my crazy self along this journey, see you guys at the top.

I would like to thank my teachers, mentors, and coaches that have guided me along this path to greatness. From my martial arts teachers, to my baseball coaches, to my school teachers, and everyone in between, thank you for you support and guidance. Special thanks to Shihan Kelly Cere, coach Brendon Toughey, coach Drew Fittry, coach Fred Tillinghast, Coach Mark Schaller, and MLB baseball player Andy Parrino just to name a few.

I would like to thank all of my personal training clients who have put their faith in me to help accomplish their goals. Without out you, Become One would not exist. Thank you for coming in and training hard with me day in and day out. But remember, the journey never ends. Your fitness journey will always be a battle. But that's why it's so great in the end. The harder the battle, the sweeter the victory! Never stop working!

Lastly I would like to thank everyone out there who's on this fitness journey with me. To all of my followers on social media who support me, the grind never ends. Press forward and climb a new rung every single day. Good things come to those who work towards something great. Take the road less traveled by and it will make all the difference! Don't forget to follow me on Twitter, Instagram, and Facebook @_become_one_ for promotions and tips.